Postpartum Depression Book for New Mom

Unveiling Motherhood, A Self-Care Guide for Navigating Secret Fears and Anxiety

Bonus: 90 days Daily Reassuring affirmations for new mothers

by

Pauline H. Byer

Copyright

Every entitlement to intellectual property is protected. Without the previous written permission of the publisher, no part of this book may be reproduced, stored in a retrieval system, or transmitted in any form or by any means, electronic, mechanical, photocopying, recording, or otherwise. Brief quotations may be used in reviews or critical articles with appropriate acknowledgment.

Disclaimer

The information contained in this book is for general informational purposes only. It is not intended to be a replacement for professional advice and should not be used as such. The author and publisher disclaim any and all liability for any injury, damage, loss, or risk incurred as a consequence, directly or indirectly, of the use and application of any content presented in this book. Readers are encouraged to seek counsel from appropriate professionals regarding their specific circumstances. The views stated in this book are the author's and do not necessarily reflect the publisher's.

About the Author

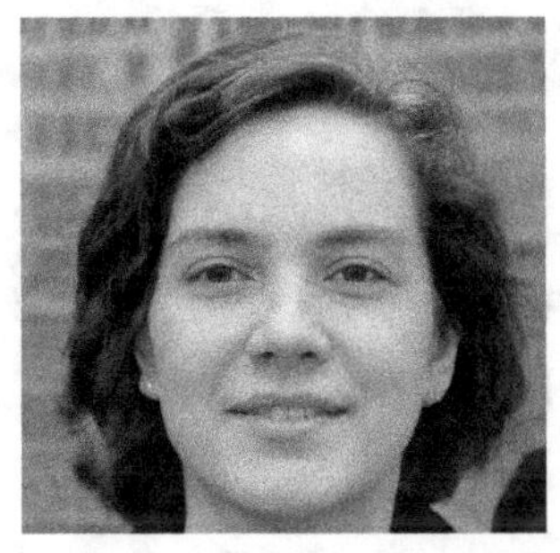 My name is Pauline H. Byer. I'm a mother, a midwife, and the driving force behind "Unveiling Motherhood." For many years, immersed in the field of childbirth and nursing, I played the dual role of mother and midwife. Each job has shaped my knowledge of the incredible journey of motherhood.

A look into my world:
Becoming a mother ignited a fire within me and an irresistible desire to uncover the complexities of life after childbirth. As a midwife, I have had the opportunity to witness the miracle of a new life being brought into this world. These experiences led me to dig deeper into postpartum depression, a topic close to my heart.

Why postpartum depression:
Postpartum depression is common in my personal and professional life. This book is my way of sharing my thoughts, stories, and practical advice to help mothers who are struggling. This is an honest attempt to bridge the gap between professional knowledge and the realities of everyday motherhood.

What I brought with me:
This book is an honest reflection of my experiences as a mother and midwife, and is based on authentic dialogue, empathy, and a deep belief in maternal resilience. This book is more than just a discussion of postpartum depression. It's also a tribute to the strength of every mother and a guide through the labyrinth of life after birth.

Our journey together:
Whether you're a new mother navigating new territory, a veteran looking for companionship, or someone interested in the complexities of postpartum depression, it's an honor to be a part

of your reading experience. Let's go on this journey together, experience the ups and downs, enjoy the chaos, and celebrate the amazing experience of motherhood.

With enthusiasm and warmth,
Byer, Pauline H.

Bonus

You can find yourself muttering, "I am a wonderful mother...I am an excellent mother..."I am a great mom," you say to yourself at 4 a.m., when your child is upset or has had a large blowout. Yes, it is correct. You ARE an excellent mother.

In reality, you probably don't get as much credit for being an excellent parent as you deserve, which is why you have to search within yourself and validate your own qualities from time to time. Affirmations about motherhood can help with this.

Choose multiple mantras that address how you're feeling each day. Perhaps you're concerned that you don't know how to care for your infant, or you're dealing with overbearing loved ones who provide unwanted advice.

Whatever the problem is, you can overcome it by taking a few deep breaths, reciting your affirmations for new moms, and viewing the situation in a new light.

These phrases do not work like magic.

They won't give you an extra hour in bed, make your postpartum body look less alien in the mirror, or stop your mother-in-law from saying "back in my day...", but they will give you the confidence boost that every new mom needs.

Daily Affirmations for New Moms

1. I am the best mother my child could have.
2. I'm doing the best I can.
3. I am surrounded by love and support for both myself and my child.
5. Accepting assistance does not imply that I am a bad mother.
6. I am growing and learning how to care for my baby every day.
7. I'm being molded into a more capable version of myself.

8. My baby does not require a perfect mother; they only require me.

9. I am qualified to care for my child.

10. I enjoy the fleeting newborn stage.

11. I value every stage my child goes through.

12. I enjoy being a mother, even on difficult days.

13. My needs are also important.

14. I look at myself through my baby's eyes rather than my own critical eyes.

15. Taking care of myself is the most effective way for me to be a present mother.

16. It is acceptable to feel overwhelmed and to require a break.

17. I can enjoy being a mother without loving every aspect of it.

18. I am thankful for my perfect child.
When I'm frustrated, I lower my standards.

19. I express my love for my baby through my actions and words.

20. I am always looking for the best way to express my love for my baby.

21. I am kind and compassionate to myself.

22. I accept the challenge of motherhood as a steep learning curve.

23. I am the person who is most familiar with my baby and their needs.

24.Taking a break from my baby is beneficial.

25. In the eyes of my child, I am an excellent mother.

26. Everything I do is for the benefit of my child.

27. I am a person apart from motherhood.

28. Motherhood is an important part of my life, but it does not define me.

29. I always make the best decisions for my child.

30. I will do better when I know better.

31. I'm leaning into this season with all of my might.

32. Motherhood is challenging at times, but I have the strength to face it.

33. As a new mother, I learn from my mistakes.

34. Learning a new skill takes time and patience, and motherhood is no exception.

35. My family is happy when I am happy.

36. My faith in my mothering abilities grows stronger by the day.

37. I serve as a positive role model for my child and other new mothers.

38. I am an inspiration to other mothers.

39. I am free to be open and honest about how I am feeling.

40. I need to take care of myself in order to be a good mother.

41. I can be inspired by other mothers while remaining true to myself.

42. I appreciate the time I get to spend with my child.

43. The most important thing is that my baby is happy and healthy.

44. I take a deep breath and let go of the situation's stress.

45. I am a quick study.

46. How other mothers raise their children has no bearing on how I raise mine.

47. Being a mother gives me a sense of purpose.

48. As a mother, I trust my intuition and instincts.

49. Other people's assessments of my parenting abilities are just that: assessments.

50. I am a blessing to my child.

51. There is a reason why my baby chose me as their mother.

52. Motherhood reveals a layer of strength within me that I was unaware of.

53. I give myself permission to rest.

54.Every day, my bond with my baby grows stronger.

55. When I am struggling, I reach out to others.

Every day, I give myself patience and grace.

57. I make a difference in the life of my child.

58. I thoroughly enjoy being a mother.

59. I am overwhelmed with gratitude and love for this wonderful life.

60. Even when I don't feel like it, I am a good mother.

61. Becoming a mother has altered my life for the better.

62. I am a self-assured and capable parent.

63. Motherhood is a gift.

64. I strive to be the best mother I can be.

65. My baby and I are intimately and divinely bonded.

66. I accept advice while listening to my inner wisdom.

67. My best is sufficient.

68. Asking for help does not imply that I am a failure.

69. Every day is a new chance to get to know my baby better.

70. I can solve any problem that comes my way.

71. Every moment presents a new opportunity for me to practice patience and kindness.

72. I, too, deserve to be taken care of.

73. I am capable of overcoming any obstacle.

74. My baby will only be this small once, so I will make the most of this brief period.

75. It's a lot of fun to see my baby grow and develop.

76. I am a caring and loving mother.

77. When I am in an uncomfortable situation, I am confident in expressing my desires.

78. I am overwhelmed by a love I had no idea existed.

79. I must prioritize rest for both myself and my child.

80. Motherhood is a practice that gets easier with time.

81. I thank my body for growing and nurturing life.

82. I am my baby's greatest source of comfort.

83. My baby seeks safety, comfort, and love from me.

84. I am the only constant in my baby's life.

85. I concentrate on what I'm doing well.

86. There are a million different ways to be a good mother.

87. It comes naturally to me to be a mother.

88. My baby and I are still getting to know each other.

89. As I learn how to be a mother, I am patient with myself.

90. I exhale stress and inhale peace.

Last Words on Affirmations for New Moms
When it all becomes too much, you don't know what's bothering your baby, or you're desperate for an uninterrupted shower, use these new mom

affirmations to remind yourself that this season is SHORT.

These newborn moments seem to last forever until they vanish in an instant, never to be seen again.

That's not to say you have to love every aspect of motherhood, but these mantras will remind you that you're tough as nails and will help you explore the sleepless nights, codependency, and poop explosions with grace.

Table of Contents

INTRODUCTION

First and foremost, congrats to new moms on your new bundle of joy. The road to motherhood is a crazy trip, and I'm delighted you've chosen this book to accompany me on it. I'm here to be your guide, confidante, and cheerleader as you navigate the ups and downs of postpartum life.

So, let's get down to business. Being a new parent is exciting, but it is also difficult. You're probably feeling a little bit of everything right now, from the beautiful moments of snuggling with your new one to the sleepless nights that make you question everything. That's perfectly OK. This book is all about stating, "I get it," confronting your worries, and providing you with some strong tactics to rock this new motherhood gig.

In the pages ahead, we'll dig into the weeds of postpartum depression, tackle the fears that every new mom has, and discuss ways to deal with those low-key worrying periods. We'll also discuss the changes your body is undergoing - no sugarcoating, just straight discussion. And, when it comes to antidepressants and postpartum depression, we'll cut through the medical language to focus on what it means for you and your baby, especially if you're nursing.

Isn't the fourth trimester like a crash course in infant boot camp?I've got your back with helpful hints to assist you get through this tempest. And we'll have some open discussions about the messy, unexpected aspects of motherhood because, let's face it, life with a newborn is anything but Pinterest-perfect.

Building a support system is critical, and we'll look at how to rely on your folks - friends, family, and even professionals - so you don't feel like you're doing it alone.This isn't a one-size-fits-all situation; it's about figuring out what works best for you and your own journey.

Okay, here's how you can use this book as a companion in this amazing adventure:

Getting Through the Unknowns: Have you ever felt like you're in unfamiliar territory? This book has your back, giving real-life stories and tips on navigating the unknowns of parenthood.

Managing Postpartum Reality: Postpartum life can be an emotional rollercoaster. We're getting into the meat of the matter - the highs, lows, and everything in between - and devising tactics to make it go more smoothly.

Dealing with Mom Anxiety: Mom anxiety exists. This book provides practical advice for dealing with the pressures that creep into your day-to-day parent life.

Self-Care Puts YOU First: Remember that'me time' everyone talks about? Yes, we're working on it. This book will help you embrace self-care because you deserve it.

Finding Your Mom Tribe: Do you feel a little lonely? Let's talk about construction. Interacting with others, and knowing it's alright to seek for assistance.

Real Talk About Motherhood: There's no fluff here, just honest discussions on the messy, beautiful, and plain difficult aspects of motherhood. We're staying true to ourselves.
Rolling with the Mom Body Changes: Your body has been through a lot, which is something to be proud of. Let's embrace the changes and own that postpartum glow together.

Early Survival Suggestions: What is the fourth trimester? It's a tornado. This book provides some practical advice to help you survive and thrive throughout your baby's early days.

Understanding Antidepressants 101: If you're on an antidepressant, we'll simplify it down for you without using medical language.

Clear, honest information about what it means for you and your child.

Empowering YOU: At the end of the day, this book is all about empowering you. It's your reminder that you're not alone, with practical skills and encouraging words to help you rock parenting with confidence, resilience, and a dash of joy. You can do it!"

So, have a seat, a warm drink (or a cold one - you've earned it), and let's speak about postpartum life. We'll face the hurdles together, enjoy the victories, and make this crazy ride a little easier. Welcome to the clan!

CHAPTER 1

Understanding Postpartum Depression

What Is Postpartum Depression?

PPD is a complicated set of physical, mental, and behavioral variations that some women experience after childbirth. According to the DSM- 5, a primer used to diagnose internal diseases, PPD is a form of major depression that begins within 4 weeks after delivery. The opinion of postpartum depression is grounded not only on the length of time between delivery and onset but on the inflexibility of the depression. Postpartum depression is linked to chemical, social, and cerebral changes that be when having a baby. The term describes a range of physical and emotional changes that numerous new mothers experience. PPD is treatable with medications and comforting words.

The chemical alterations include a quick decline in hormone levels following delivery. The precise relationship between this decline and depression is still unknown. But it is known that during pregnancy, the levels of estrogen and progesterone, the female reproductive hormones, increase tenfold. They then fall precipitously following delivery. These hormone levels return to pre-pregnancy levels three days after a woman delivers birth.

Aside from these physical changes, having a baby creates social and psychological changes that increase the chances of depression. The majority of new mothers have "baby blues" after giving birth. One in every ten of these women will experience a more severe and long-lasting depression after giving birth. Postpartum psychosis affects approximately one in every 1,000 women.

Not even dads are exempted. According to research, one out of every ten new fathers experiences depression during the first year of their child's life.

Types of Postpartum Depression
Three terms are used to describe the mood changes that women can experience after giving birth:

•As many as 70% of women have **"baby blues"** in the days following childbirth. You may have abrupt mood fluctuations, such as feeling very pleased and then quite depressed. You may cry for no apparent cause and experience feelings of impatience, crankiness, restlessness, anxiety, loneliness, and sadness. The baby blues can continue for a few hours or up to two weeks after birth. Baby blues are usually not serious enough to warrant medical attention. Joining a new parents' support group or conversing with other moms can often assist.

•**Postpartum depression (PPD)** can strike days, weeks, or even months after giving birth. PPD can occur with the birth of any child, not just the first. You can experience sensations comparable to the baby blues, such as melancholy, despair, anxiety, and crankiness, but much more intensely. PPD frequently prevents you from doing the things you need to do on a daily basis. When your capacity to function is impaired, you should consult with a health care practitioner, such as your OB/GYN or primary care physician. This doctor can assess you for depression symptoms and develop a treatment plan for you. If you do not get treatment for PPD, your symptoms may worsen. Although PPD is a serious disease, it is treatable with medication and treatment.

•**Postpartum psychosis** is a severe mental disease that can occur in new mothers. This sickness can strike swiftly, frequently during the first three months following childbirth. Women can experience auditory hallucinations (hearing things that aren't actually happening, such as a person talking) and delusions (strongly believing things that are clearly unreasonable). Visual hallucinations (seeing objects that aren't there) are rarer. Other symptoms include inability to sleep, agitation and anger, pacing, restlessness, and unusual feelings and actions. Women suffering from postpartum psychosis require immediate treatment and almost invariably require medication. Women are sometimes admitted to the hospital because they are in danger of injuring themselves or others.

Is It Postpartum Depression or 'Baby Blues'?
Having a child is a significant adjustment in your life. You undoubtedly anticipate to be happy and proud of your new family member, but many mothers are grumpy and stressed instead

It's natural to experience this for a short period of time. Hormone levels decline after giving delivery, which affects your mood. Because your newborn is waking up at unusual hours, you're probably not getting enough sleep. That in itself may upset you. You could simply be worried about caring for your baby, which can lead you to experience stress that you haven't before encountered.

It's Not Just You

You are not the first mother to experience these phases of emotions. Approximately eighty percent of new mothers experience "baby blues," which are short-term emotional swings triggered by all of the changes that come with having a new baby. These feelings are common when the baby is only 2 or 3 days old, but they should pass by the time your baby is 1 or 2 weeks old.

If your sadness stays longer than that, or worsens instead of improving, you may be suffering from postpartum depression. It is more powerful and lasts longer than the baby blues, which afflict approximately 10% of moms. If you've previously had depression or if it runs in your family, you're more likely to suffer from postpartum depression.

How can you tell if you have the baby blues or postpartum depression?

You may have baby blues if:

•Your mood swings from cheerful to sad quickly. One minute, you're pleased of your work as a new mother. The next thing you know, you're weeping because you don't think you're up to the task.

•You're fatigued and don't want to eat or take care of yourself.

•You're irritated, overwhelmed, and worried.

You may have Postpartum depression if:

•You are always depressed, unhappy, worthless, or lonely, and you cry frequently.

•You don't think you're doing a good job as a new mother.

•You aren't connecting with your child.

•Because of your tremendous despair, you are unable to eat, sleep, or care for your newborn.

•You may experience panic and anxiousness episodes.

Overview of Postpartum Depression (PPD)

The arrival of a newborn can bring about a wide range of strong emotions, from excitement and happiness to dread and anxiety. However, it can also lead to something unexpected: depression.

Most new mothers suffer from postpartum "baby blues" following childbirth, which include mood changes, weeping episodes, anxiety, and problems sleeping. Baby blues typically begin within the first two to three days of birth and can linger for up to two weeks.

However, some new mothers suffer from postpartum depression, a more severe and long-lasting form of depression. It's also known as peripartum depression because it can begin during pregnancy and last beyond childbirth. Postpartum psychosis is a rare serious mood illness that can occur after childbirth.

Postpartum depression is neither a defect nor a character flaw. Sometimes it's just a side effect of giving birth. If you suffer postpartum depression, getting the right help in time can help you handle your symptoms and bond with your baby.

Mother-infant relationship

Postpartum depression can disrupt normal mother-infant attachment and have a negative impact both short and long term on child development. Mothers suffering from postpartum depression may be inconsistent with childcare. Feeding routines, sleep routines, and health maintenance are examples of childcare discrepancies.

Postpartum psychosis arises in 1 to 2 out of every 1,000 cases of postpartum depression. Infanticide may occur in these cases, as well as in women who have a history of previous psychiatric hospitalizations. Postpartum depression is one of the primary causes of the annual reported infanticide incidence rate of roughly 8 per 100,000 births in the United States.

Postpartum depression can affect children, according to research published in the American Journal of Obstetrics and Gynecology. If a mother's postpartum depression remains untreated, it can have a negative impact on her children. When a child is young, these issues can include excessive crying (colic) and irregular sleeping patterns. These issues can have a cyclical effect, meaning they can aggravate the mother's postpartum depression and potentially lead to the mother experiencing postpartum depression again. These cyclical impacts can have an impact on the mother's ability to sustain her relationship with her baby. Breastfeeding cessation is one example, as are negative emotions such as withdrawal, disengagement, and even hate. If a mother develops an antagonistic relationship with her child, it can lead to extreme events such as infanticide.

Postpartum depression, as the kid grows older, can cause anomalies in cognitive processes, actions, and emotions. In addition to these abnormalities, children who grew up in the presence of postpartum depression are more likely to acquire aggressive inclinations.

Postpartum Depression Causes and Risk Factors

If you experience PPD, it is not due of anything you did wrong. Experts believe it happens for a variety of causes, which vary from person to person. Some factors that can increase the likelihood of postpartum depression include:

•Age at the period of pregnancy (the younger you are, the greater your chances are).
•Uncertainty regarding the pregnancy
•Kids (the more you have, the more likely you will be depressed later in your subsequent pregnancy)

•A history of mood disorders in the family

•Experiencing a highly stressful situation, such as a job loss or a health problem
•Having a child who has special needs or health issues
•Restricted social support
•Alone living
•Marital discord

There is no one cause of postpartum depression, however the following physical and emotional factors may play a role:

•**Hormones.** The substantial decline in estrogen and progesterone after giving birth could be a factor. Other hormones generated by the thyroid gland may also fall sharply, leaving you weary, sluggish, and sad.

•**Inadequate sleep.** When you're sleep-deprived and overwhelmed, you may struggle to deal with even simple issues.

•**Anxiety.** You could be concerned about your abilities to care for a newborn.

•**Self-image.** You may feel less beautiful, question your identity, or believe you've lost control of your life. Any of these causes can contribute to postpartum depression.

Postpartum Depression Complications

Untreated postpartum depression can impair your capacity to bond with your newborn and affect the entire family:

•**You.** Untreated postpartum depression can linger for months or even years, progressing to a chronic depressive condition. Even with treatment, postpartum depression can increase your risk of future depression episodes.

•**The father of the child.** When a new mother suffers from depression, the father is more likely to suffer from depression as well.

•**Children.** Children of moms suffering from postpartum depression are more likely to have sleeping and feeding problems, cry more than usual, and experience delays in language development.

CHAPTER 2

Recognizing signs and symptoms

PPD symptoms might appear at any time during the first year after giving birth.Postpartum depression is often diagnosed after signs and symptoms have persisted for a minimum of two weeks.

Emotional
•Continual sorrow, anxiety, or a "empty" mood
•Extreme mood swings
•Frustration, impatience, agitation, and wrath
•A sense of powerlessness or hopelessness
•Guilt, shame, and a sense of worthlessness
•A lack of self-esteem
•Anxiety, emptiness
•Exhaustion
•The inability to be consoled
•Difficulties bonding with the baby
•Feeling inadequate to care for the infant

•Contemplations of self-harm or suicide

Behavioral
•A lack of interest or enjoyment in typical activities
•Inadequate libido
•Appetite changes
•Fatigue, low energy, and motivation
•Inadequate self-care
•Withdrawal from social activities
•Insomnia or sleeping excessively
•Concerns about killing oneself, one's child, or one's partner

Neurobiology
Functional magnetic resonance imaging (fMRI) studies show differences in brain activity between moms with and without postpartum depression. When compared to healthy controls, mothers with PPD have less activity in the left frontal lobe and more activity in the right frontal lobe. They also have reduced connection between important brain areas such as the anterior cingulate cortex, dorsal lateral prefrontal

cortex, amygdala, and hippocampus. When prompted by non-infant emotional stimuli, brain activity disparities between sad and nondepressed moms became more significant. Depressed moms have increased brain activity in the right amygdala in response to non-infant emotional signals and decreased connection between the amygdala and the right insular cortex. Recent research has also found that women with ADHD have reduced activity in the anterior cingulate cortex, striatum, orbitofrontal cortex, and insula.

Importance of early intervention

It's not always clear how postpartum depression will manifest itself. Most women's symptoms go away on their own without therapy, but after a year, 20% of them still experience substantial depressive symptoms.

Screening for postpartum depression risk is crucial since the condition of the woman, her child, and her family as a whole is all impacted by postpartum depression. Nowadays, the majority of obstetricians use a screening instrument of some kind during the postpartum examination. Studies have indicated that many women with postpartum depression are ashamed of their symptoms and fear the social stigma attached to the diagnosis, which makes screening crucial.

Postpartum depression can present with a variety of symptoms, but common ones include:
•disturbances in sleep
• Anxiety
•Aggression
• having a sense of overwhelm
•an obsession with the health or nutrition of the infant

Postpartum depression is diagnosed on the basis of more than simply the existence of these symptoms. Some of them may be typical, particularly following a trying and restless night of taking care of a newborn. The diagnosis of postpartum depression depends on the severity of the symptoms and how they interfere with the woman's capacity to cope and adjust to her environment.

Treating postpartum depression

Treatment and recovery time vary based on the severity of your depression and your specific needs. If you have an underactive thyroid or an underlying condition, your doctor may treat it or refer you to a specialist. Your health care provider may also refer you to a mental health specialist.

Doctors in their research emphasized the significance of early treatment and support for women who are at risk of postpartum depression, even those who have mild symptoms but do not fulfill the exact criteria for a formal diagnosis of postpartum depression. According to research, supportive and psychological care provided immediately after birth can reduce an at-risk woman's likelihood of developing postpartum depression. Interventions that reduce feelings of loneliness and give emotional support are critical; examples include:

•House calls
•peer help via the phone
•Interpersonal counseling

When a new mother is diagnosed with postpartum depression, it is critical that she receives the care she requires. The intensity of a woman's symptoms and how she responds to the intervention determine the recommended treatment.The approach for postpartum women with mild symptoms is quite similar to the preventative efforts for at-risk mothers. These are some examples:

•psychological therapies addressing new mother support
•Support organizations
•nurse visits at home

Treatment for women with moderate symptoms or mild symptoms who did not react to the initial intervention comprises of formal psychotherapy alone or in combination with an antidepressant drug. If the lady wishes or if getting to therapy is problematic, antidepressants can be administered alone.

The safety of antidepressant drugs while breastfeeding is a common worry. Selective serotonin reuptake inhibitors (SSRIs) are the first-line treatment for postpartum depression, and only trace levels are present in breast milk.

Experts generally concur that mothers do not need to discontinue nursing, despite the lack of long-term research about the effects of antidepressants on breastfed babies. However "clinicians should support women in their choice not to breastfeed when difficulties in the breastfeeding process, or lack of sleep, are perpetuating depressive symptoms." This is an essential issue.

Early intervention is essential for both the prevention and effective treatment of postpartum depression. After having a child, women may not recognize that they are depressed or may recognize that they are having difficulties but feel too ashamed to get treatment. This is the reason screening all new mothers is crucial. Women should be urged to disclose their postpartum depression symptoms.

Lifestyle and home remedies

In addition to professional treatment, you can take steps to supplement your treatment plan and speed up your recovery.

•**Make healthier lifestyle choices.**Include physical activity, such as a stroll with your baby, and other forms of exercise in what you do every day. Try to get plenty of rest. Take healthy meals and avoid alcohol.

•**Shun every unrealistic expectation.** Do not put too much pressure on yourself to accomplish everything. Lower your expectations for the perfect household. Do what you can and let go of the remaining.

•**Make time just for yourself.** Take some time for yourself and leave the house. This could mean asking a partner to care for the baby or hiring a sitter. Engage in an enjoyable activity, such as a hobby or entertainment. You could also set aside some time alone with your partner or friends.

•**Ask for assistance.**Try to open up to those closest to you and tell them you need help. Accept someone's offer to babysit. If you can sleep, take a nap, go see a movie, or meet up with friends for coffee. You may also benefit from seeking assistance with parenting skills, which can include caregiving techniques for improving your baby's sleep and soothing fussing and crying.

Remember that caring for your baby also means caring for yourself.

Getting ready for your appointment
Following your initial consultation, your physician might suggest that you see a mental

health professional who can collaborate with you to develop an appropriate treatment plan. Seek the assistance of a reliable friend or family member to attend your appointment in order to aid in your memory of all the information covered.

Prior to your meeting, jot down the following:
•What symptoms, and how long, have you been having?
•Your entire medical history, including any physical or mental illnesses, such as depression.
•Every medication you take, including over-the-counter and prescription drugs, vitamins, herbal remedies, and other supplements, as well as the dosages.
•Questions to put to your provider.

Questions to put to your provider may include the following:
•What's the diagnosis I have?
•Which therapies are most likely to benefit me?
•What adverse effects might the treatments you recommend have?

•How much and when do you think the treatment will help my symptoms?

•Is it safe to take the medication you're recommending while nursing.

•For what duration will I require treatment?

•What adjustments to my lifestyle can help me control my symptoms?

•How frequently should I go in for follow-up?

•Do I have a higher chance of developing other mental health issues?

•If I have another child, am I going to have this condition again?

•If I have another child, is there a way to stop it from happening again?

•Are there any printed materials available for me to obtain? Which internet sites would you suggest I check out?

During your appointment, feel free to ask any additional questions you may have.

What to anticipate from your doctor
You might be asked certain questions by your mental health or medical professional, like:

•What symptoms do you have, and when did they first appear?

•Has the quality or severity of your symptoms changed over time?

•Do your symptoms make it difficult for you to take care of your child?

•Do you and your child feel as bonded as you thought?

•When it's time to wake up, can you get out of bed and go to sleep when you can?

•What would you say about your level of energy?

•Has your appetite changed since then?

•What is the frequency of your anxiety, irritability, or anger?

•Have you considered hurting your child or yourself?

•How much help do you get to take care of your child?

•Do you have any other significant stressors in your life, such as relationship or money issues?

•Have you received a diagnosis for any other illnesses?

•Have you ever had a mental health diagnosis, such as bipolar disorder or depression? If so, which kind of care was most beneficial?

Further questions may be asked by your provider in light of your needs, symptoms, and answers. Making the most of your appointment will be facilitated by being ready for questions.

CHAPTER 3

Real Fears Every New Mom Faces

Being in charge of a newborn is one of the most incredible—and terrifying—task you can accomplish. But here come the good news: you're not alone in your concerns. That's why we interviewed real moms to find out what their main concerns were, and then conducted research to put things in context. Here are the top fears that new moms have and why they aren't worth worrying about.

1. Am I doing all possible to reduce the risk of SIDS (sudden infant death syndrome)?

To feel better about it, do the following: The most common dread of new parents is sudden infant death syndrome (SIDS), commonly known as crib death since it frequently occurs during sleep. In fact, more than one mother admitted to having accidentally woken up to check on her napping baby to make sure they were still breathing. While there is no proven cause for SIDS (the mysterious death of a seemingly healthy baby under the age of 12 months), experts do know that some conditions put babies at risk. One of the most common is putting a baby to sleep facedown on their stomach or side. In reality, the prevalence of SIDS in the United States reduced by 53% over the next decade after the American Academy of Pediatrics (AAP) launched its "Back to Sleep" campaign. Always put your infant to sleep on their back, as recommended by the American Academy of Pediatrics. You should also put your infant on a hard mattress and keep any soft objects out of the sleeping area (such as cushions, stuffed animals, loose bedding, or crib bumpers). Other recommendations include practicing room sharing (but not bed sharing), putting your baby to sleep with a pacifier if they'll take it, and making sure they don't become too hot while sleeping. Finally, ensure that your child has all of the necessary immunizations—this is crucial for a variety of reasons, but it is also related with a 50% lower incidence of SIDS.

2. What if I don't know how to breastfeed?

To feel better about it, do the following: To be honest, it may take some time for you and your baby to get into the habit of nursing. But the good news is that there are plenty of services available if you need assistance (and many women do). If you are concerned, check with a lactation consultant before giving birth and inquire whether your hospital will have one available after delivery. Alternatively, contact a mom buddy who has been there and done that. "The best thing a woman can do to prepare for breastfeeding before the baby comes is to watch babies nurse," says international board-certified lactation consultant Leigh Anne O'Connor. Contact a breastfeeding support organization in your region (La Leche League is an excellent resource) and attend a demonstration or devote an afternoon watching your bestie in action.

(Remember, there's plenty of proof that it's perfectly fine if you can't nurse.)

3. What if my child develops a flat head?

To feel better about it, do the following: Flat head syndrome (plagiocephaly) occurs when a flat patch forms on the back or side of a baby's head. And, to be honest, it's fairly frequent (one research discovered that over half of all infants aged 7 to 12 weeks had plagiocephaly). But don't worry, mama; this normally works itself out. (How many adults do you notice walking around with their heads bowed? There aren't many.) However, there are several simple strategies to avoid flat head syndrome, such as rotating your baby's head position during sleep and providing plenty of supervised tummy time. Your doctor can ensure that everything is developing normally if you keep up with your baby's well visits.

4. What if I accidently open the scab on the baby's umbilical stump while cleaning it?

How to feel better about it: Pediatricians usually advise against touching it. Instead, simply keep the region dry and expose it to air as often as possible to help dry up the scab (you can tuck the diaper down to prevent covering it and use kimono tops instead of onesies to avoid covering it). Avoid using the bathtub until the scab has gone off (this should happen within a week or two), and instead take sponge baths. You can do it.

5. What if my infant becomes overheated? What if she gets cold?

To feel better about it, do the following: One mother told us that she was obsessed with temperature for the first few weeks of her daughter's existence. ("Is she overheated? Is it too cold? "Have I got enough layers on her?") The recommended temperature for the baby's room is between 68°F and 72°F (20°C to 22°C), according to experts. When in doubt, follow physician Michel Cohen's advice: "The perfect temperature for Lucy's room is room temperature." It shouldn't be too hot or too cold. To put it another way, whatever works for you works for her." Translation? Don't overthink things. (However, if you're truly concerned, invest in a digital thermometer to keep the room at a reasonable temperature.) "You can take Lucy out in frigid winter temperatures," Dr. Cohen adds of the wide outdoors. Unlike older children, newborns can be easily bundled up. Heat, on the other hand, is good; recall, Lucy lived in a kind of terrarium for nine months, with a minimum temperature of 97 degrees and no air conditioning.In other words, don't worry about it.

6. What if my baby is delayed in development?

To feel better about it, do the following:Here's one thing you shouldn't do: Don't compare your child to other children. Your cousin's month-old has begun to roll over, but your four-month-old is still turtling on his back? Not only is that perfectly OK, but it also means nothing (sorry, but this does not guarantee your child a spot at Harvard). Each infant is unique and develops at his or her own rate. That's not to imply milestones should be ignored, but don't be concerned if your micro doesn't meet them—consider them general guidelines rather than hard and fast laws. Another thing to keep in mind is that these milestones are actually ranges (for example, a child could begin walking at any time between 9 and 16 months). But, if you're worried about something, talk to your pediatrician (who will almost certainly tell you it's nothing to worry about).

7. What if my infant is not eating enough?

To feel better about it, do the following: According to the American Academy of Pediatrics, you should breastfeed your baby every two to three hours during the day and every four hours at night throughout the first month, even if you have to wake him up to eat. If you are formula feeding, your newborn will consume two to three ounces of formula per feeding (every three to four hours throughout the first few weeks). How do you know whether she is getting enough? The devil is hiding in the diapers. According to Kelly Mom, you should expect at least five or six wet diapers each day, as well as three or four poopy diapers per day, during the first six weeks. Weight gain is a further indicator. According to the American Pregnancy Association, most babies will gain five to seven ounces each week for the first few months.

Common fears and anxieties during the postpartum period

What is postpartum anxiety?

Postpartum generalized anxiety is characterized by an illogical dread or exaggerated worry that something is wrong, and it typically involves worrying all day, every day, about a variety of issues. It's similar to normal anxiety, but it's more intimately associated with having a baby and being a parent.

Many new mothers have been taught that melancholy and depression after having a baby are common and can be caused by the baby blues or postpartum depression. However, not every new mom is aware that feeling excessively nervous or afraid, or even having panic episodes, is almost as common. In reality, postpartum anxiety affects 10 to 15% of new mothers, and half of those who have postpartum depression also have postpartum anxiety.

What are the symptoms of postpartum anxiety?

Postpartum anxiety can cause the following symptoms in a mother:

•Fear or a sense of impending peril

•Thoughts that race

•A constant sense of dread, as if something terrible is about to happen.

•Extreme concern for the baby's health, development, or safety

•A crushing sense of burden, stress, and worry about one's capacity to be a decent parent

•A chronic attack of the jitters or an anxious state

•Insomnia or difficulty falling or staying asleep, despite being weary

•Changes in heart rate and respiration, such as an elevated heart rate, rapid breathing, and/or chest pain, particularly if the anxiety manifests as panic attacks

•Dizziness

•Nausea

•Shaking

•Hot flushes and/or chills

What causes postpartum anxiety?
Although there is no single cause of postpartum anxiety, a number of variables can raise the likelihood of having the condition:

•Hormonal shifts after childbirth – For some mothers, hormonal swings can have a bigger impact on overall mood and anxiety than for other women.

•Inadequate rest

•The anxiety that comes with caring for a tiny, new, helpless newborn.

•Changes in relationships that can occur as a result of a baby's birth

•Social pressure on new mothers, as well as their own expectations of being "perfect"

•Personality type – moms who are "type A," very sensitive, or easily anxious are more likely to experience postpartum anxiety.

•Having a family or personal history of mental disorders.

•A history of panic and/or anxiety attacks

•A history of miscarriage or stillbirth

•Having a premature baby or a baby with medical problems

How long does postpartum anxiety last?
There is no set timetable for postpartum anxiety, but the good news is that it is not permanent. Recovery duration can vary depending on how quickly a mother receives care. Moderate to severe anxiety might linger indefinitely if left untreated.

CHAPTER 4

Normalizing concerns for new moms

What are some misconceptions about postpartum depression?

In my experience as a Midwife, some mothers are unaware of their symptoms, while others are aware but may be scared to speak up due to stigma, the impression of neediness, or an inability to cope. So, what are the myths regarding postpartum depression?

Unfortunately, the stigma surrounding PPD has resulted in numerous prevalent misconceptions regarding the disorder, the most destructive of which is that PPD is merely a character flaw or weakness. PPD is sometimes dismissed as "baby blues," a less serious condition that affects up to 80% of new moms. While moms suffering the baby blues may experience symptoms such as mood swings, anxiety, melancholy, and insomnia, the effects usually subside within two weeks.

In reality, mental health issues are the biggest cause of pregnancy-related mortality, surpassing hemorrhage and heart disorders. As many as 52% of these maternal deaths occur up to a year after childbirth, emphasizing the importance of new moms having access to comprehensive and ongoing mental health care following childbirth. Many new mothers may not seek therapy because they are frightened of being labeled incompetent or unfit if they are unaware that PPD is one of the most serious and prevalent medical problems of pregnancy.

Many people believe that a diagnosis of PPD must occur within the first few days or weeks of childbirth. In actuality, PPD can show up to a year later and can even begin during pregnancy, which is why the ideal term for the disorder is peripartum depression.

If a patient recovers from PPD after having their first child, they may believe they are safe for future pregnancies. In reality, a diagnosis of PPD raises a patient's chance of subsequent pregnancies by 30%.

PPD is usually assumed to be an illness that only new moms face, but approximately 10% of new fathers also experience PPD as a result of hormonal changes, new relationship dynamics, and increased feelings of pressure or guilt connected with parenthood. Adoptive parents might be affected by the advent of a new child, with 10-32% developing post-adoption depression syndrome.

The importance of plan sponsor support for postpartum depression

It is be noted that if PPD is not treated, it might lead to:

•Poor adherence to care and worsening of pre-existing medical conditions

•Violence in relationships, separation, and divorce

•Decreased productivity, weariness, and loss of concentration
•Increased usage of tobacco, alcohol, and drugs
•Neglect and abuse of children
•Postpartum psychosis, which, if left untreated, can lead to infanticide, violence, or suicide.

PPD and its associated symptoms can cost up to $14.2 billion per year, with an average cost of almost $32,000 per untreated mother-child pair. Maintaining solid support networks at work, as well as providing extensive maternal leave policies and benefits, can empower new parents to care for themselves and their children when they are most vulnerable.

Access to affordable treatment is crucial, especially as PPD affects more than half of low-income women, and low income is a factor that might lead to inequities in postpartum care utilization. It is also critical for plan sponsors to put in place measures that encourage new moms to begin their ongoing care as early as possible in their pregnancy journey. Prenatal care use is the best predictor of postpartum care utilization and, ultimately, the best approach to manage a PPD diagnosis.

Moreover, individuals suffering from PPD should be aware that it is a common, treatable disease with several resources. To achieve full recovery, it is critical to seek support and have regular appointments with a postpartum care team.

Strategies for managing fears

Strategy 1: Develop a higher tolerance for uncertainty.

According to research, most people who worry excessively have trouble dealing with ambiguity. That is, whenever they are unsure of something, even if it is as simple as whether there will be enough parking at the doctor's office, they are likely to be concerned.

However, because no one can anticipate the future, practically everything in life is uncertain. If uncertainty is causing a lot of your problems, the best way to deal with it is to get more comfortable with not knowing everything all of the time. When you worry, you are attempting to achieve the alternative option, which is to have 100% certainty. However, you are already aware that this strategy is not particularly effective. If it were, you wouldn't have any need to be anxious!

So, how can you learn how to live with unpredictability? The best solution is to change your behavior and appear "as if" you are at ease with it.

Some strategies for increasing tolerance for uncertainty include:
•Resisting the urge to weigh your baby every week unless your doctor has instructed you to do so.
•Without a medical reason, discontinuing the diary of all the baby's feeding, wet diapers, and poopy diapers.
•Following the health department's newborn vaccination protocols without performing any Internet research.

•Taking the baby to the grocery store without a list.

•Before leaving the house, only once check the diaper bag contents.

•Requesting that your partner bathe and dress the baby while you go for a stroll.

Strategy 2: If you are concerned about present problems, do what you can to remedy them.

Some situations are directly under your control. You can, for example, budget to manage your funds or determine which stroller to purchase. The greatest strategy to deal with current issues is to concentrate on what you can do to assist address the problem.

When people worry, they believe they are fixing problems. Most of the time, the reverse is true. When you worry, you are mentally going over a problem. However, problem solving requires action rather than rumination. It entails getting out of your own brain and doing something about it. Worriers frequently become so concerned that they postpone tackling the problem or procrastinate.

Taking action to remedy a problem will most likely reduce your anxiety. You have one fewer item to worry about for every problem you solve.

Strategy 3: Create a concern script for worrying about hypothetical events.
Concerns concerning hypothetical situations, unlike existing concerns, cannot usually be addressed through immediate action. For example, activities taken today will not alleviate your concerns about your infant acquiring an ailment later in life. Some things are simply beyond your ability to control. Writing a worry script is the finest strategy for dealing with hypothetical fears.

A concern script is not the same as just putting down your anxieties. The goal is to express your concerns in writing as if they were true and to elicit an emotional response. You will write about your concerns and what you are concerned about. For example, if you are concerned that your child gets autism, you could include in your worry script your concerns about recognizing autism symptoms in your infant, getting him or her diagnosed, and what might happen, such as lifelong difficulty managing a challenged child.

A worry script allows you to experience, rather than avoid, the negative emotions linked with your fears and worries. Although this will be uncomfortable at first, research suggests that confronting your anxieties in this manner reduces anxiety and worries over time. A concern script also assists you in visualizing your dreaded consequence rather than thinking about it in "fuzzy" or imprecise manners.

CHAPTER 5

Navigating Mild Anxiety

A "Mild" anxiety

Almost no one dealing with chronic anxiety would describe it as "mild." Most people experiencing subjectively mild anxiety are unlikely to believe they have anxiety at all. But what exactly is mild anxiety, and are there any easier ways to overcome it.

However, regardless of the results, anxiety is always difficult to deal with. Anxiety is always a struggle, no matter how mild or severe it is; otherwise, you would not be aware that you had it.

It is essential to remember that if anxiety is affecting your quality of life, it should be treated. Don't pay attention to terms like "mild" or "severe." If you suffer from anxiety and it bothers you, seek treatment.

How to Describe Mild Anxiety?

Mild anxiety is anxiety that can be managed with no additional techniques. By "manageable," we do not mean that it is easily removed. We're saying you can still get through your day without panicking, have a social life, and even find hobbies and activities enjoyable. You might even think positively about the future.

Mild anxiety occurs when you have irritating symptoms that don't seem to go away but don't control you. For example:

•You have steady worries, but you can usually ignore them.

•You may feel nervous, nauseated, shaky, or sweaty, but these symptoms do not impair your health.

•You do not experience panic attacks or become so overwhelmed by your anxiety that you begin to fear it.

Mild anxiety is similar to moderate anxiety, with the exception that it rarely or never reaches the point of being truly overwhelming. It's more of a hassle that you can't seem to control, with occasional bouts of severity that remind you that you have to deal with it.

Many anxiety disorders can be mild, too. Panic attacks are rarely mild, but there is mild obsessive-compulsive disorder, mild generalized anxiety disorder, and mild phobias. Post-traumatic stress disorder is more difficult to diagnose, and mild social anxiety is relatively common and rarely considered a serious disorder.

All Anxiety Should Be Treated

If your anxiety is "mild," it does not mean you should ignore it. Most anxiety starts out mild before worsening as you get older, especially if you don't treat it. Furthermore, anxiety is such a treatable condition that those who tolerate mild anxiety simply because it is not severe enough are jeopardizing their quality of life.

Mild anxiety should always be addressed. Even anxiety that is not classified as an anxiety disorder warrants attention. Anxiety is not a good emotion. If you were always sad or angry, you would seek help; there is no reason why you should not seek the same level of assistance if you suffer from mild anxiety.

How to handle Mild Anxiety

The only advantage of mild anxiety over more severe anxiety is that those with mild anxiety are less likely to fear their anxiety symptoms than those with severe anxiety. This is beneficial because severe anxiety attacks can interfere with your treatment in ways that mild anxiety attacks should not.

Simple lifestyle changes may help you manage mild anxiety. Consider the following:

Exercise regularly.

Even if you don't do anything else, make sure to exercise on a regular basis. Exercise is an effective and valuable mental health tool. Endorphins are released during exercise, calming the entire body. It depletes adrenaline, which is released during anxiety, and may burn away stress hormones. It relaxes your muscles, reducing anxiety symptoms, and it reduces overall physical stress, which studies have shown can also reduce mental stress. Exercise is the most important thing you can do to alleviate mild anxiety.

Sleep, diet, etc.

While not as beneficial as exercise, overall healthy living is important. Remember that real science has shown that a stressed body can cause anxiety and negative thoughts. Your mind and body work together closely. Getting enough sleep and eating healthier can significantly reduce physical and mental stress, making coping with anxiety much easier.

Learn relaxation techniques

Counseling can still be extremely beneficial for people with mild anxiety. However, for those who want to avoid therapy, basic relaxation techniques may be sufficient. Begin by practicing deep breathing, visualization, and progressive muscle relaxation. Make sure you commit to them for at least two months. Contrary to popular belief, relaxation exercises do not work immediately. They only work if you become accustomed to performing them without overthinking the actions.

Differentiating between normal worries and anxiety

Occasional worries or moments of stress constitute a normal aspect of parenting. Abnormal anxiety occurs when those worries aren't rooted in a realistic fear or they begin to control your actions.

What is the distinction between normal worry and anxiety? This can be the million-dollar question for mothers who are on edge, stressed, nervous, or simply on high alert.

Many mothers wonder if they are experiencing abnormal anxiety, general stress, or normal worry. Because they can all appear similar, it can be difficult to tell the difference.A good way to figure out whether your experiences are "normal" is to ask yourself, "Is this becoming a problem in my life?"

It's normal to be worried. Every parent occasionally worries about their children's well-being. Consider how natural that is: there are more things to keep on your radar, more potential threats to assess, and you are responsible for taking reasonable precautions to protect your children. Occasional worries or moments of stress are a normal part of parenthood.

However, abnormal anxiety occurs when those worries are not based on a realistic fear or when they begin to control your actions and daily life. If you're unsure if your anxiety is excessive, this guide can clarify what's normal and what isn't.

Normal worry looks like this:
If your fears or worries match the descriptions below, you're probably in the "normal" zone.

•The problem you're working on is an attempt to solve a current situation.
When a threat or real problem arises, it is natural to worry about it. If, for example, you are considering appropriate actions in response to your child being bullied at school, that is a normal concern. The stress is justified because the situation is real and has an impact on you.

•You have some control over your worry cycle.
Are you able to separate yourself from whatever is stressing you out, or does it take up all of your mental space? **If** you have some emotional control over the circumstance, what you're feeling is still within the usual range of worry. If you can think about it but then put it aside to have dinner with your family or answer a phone call from your sister, that's a positive indicator.

•These concerns are a result of a specific trigger.

What happened before you were worried? When there is a definite cause or trigger, the subsequent thoughts are usually a natural response.For example, if you see a car driving significantly above the speed limit immediately outside your house where your children play, it's natural to be concerned about an accident and relocate your children to a safer location.

•You don't spend the majority of your time in a panic loop.

If you can keep your thoughts in check without losing control, you're likely feeling regular worry rather than more serious anxiety. Ask yourself: am I looking at a problem realistically and without exaggerating it, or am I focusing on unlikely worst-case scenarios? If it is the former, you are doing well.

Signs you could be dealing with abnormal anxiety:

There is a difference between normal, healthy worry and anxiety that is unproductive and unhealthy. These are the warning signs that anxiety is present.

•You're seeking to lower overall uncertainty.
A lot of unhealthy anxiety stems from a need for control. Are you continually attempting to handle situations over which you have no control? That is impossible to achieve. That only adds to the anxiety and overwhelm. While it may appear to be beneficial, it is not.

•There is no specific cause; you are simply worried out of habit.
There's a considerable difference between noticing something distressing or receiving a stressful message and then reacting emotionally to it. However, if you are constantly anxious, regardless of whether or not something has triggered that concern, you may be dealing with anxiety that is no longer considered normal. Do you wake up worried? Do you have anxiety spikes at various periods for no apparent reason?

•Your thoughts are unlikely to be focused.

It's one thing to be concerned about a child's skinned knee and then sterilize and bandage the wound. It's another thing to presume it will become infected, to constantly check the injury, and to keep your child from riding her bike as a precaution. To distinguish between healthy worry and unhealthy anxiety, ask yourself, "Is what I'm fearing logical and realistic, or is this scenario in my mind unlikely?"

•The anxiety is interfering with daily living.

When your activities change in an attempt to prevent or avoid whatever is generating the anxiety, this is one of the most telling symptoms that a regular, understandable dread has gone over into abnormal anxiety. If your daily life, routine, or relationships are being jeopardized as a result of whatever is causing you stress, this is no longer normal, and you do not have to live with or accept it.

CHAPTER 6

Coping mechanisms for mild anxiety

Here are some tips and reminders for soon-to-be and new moms on how to manage anxiety:

1. Anxiety at first is entirely normal and evolutionary significant.

You should be a little nervous at first. Check to see if the baby is breathing on a regular basis. You want to look into all kinds of questions. For mothers, this is a rite of passage. So many moms talk about breastfeeding or staying up late reading "how often should the baby eat?"

2. Your level of anxiousness will fluctuate over time. While I was initially concerned about my child's safety, I no longer worry about some of the other issues that used to worry me. When I began sleeping for extended periods of time at night, I began to worry about other things, such as the never-ending mounds of dishes and laundry. I recall doing six loads of laundry in

one day and not believing it. That was the day I realized we had progressed from safety concerns to a higher level of concern for the proper operation of the house. It's very normal to be concerned about one set of difficulties at one stage of growth and another set of concerns at another.

3. Identify one or two ways to exercise self-care every day, even if it's extremely difficult. I was adamant about taking a shower every day. Not all new moms have the time or stamina to take a shower every day, but this was a must for me. For some mothers, it could be an hour a day to do something for themselves. It doesn't matter what it is or how long it takes; find that one item that will return you to some sense of normalcy. As my child has grown older, I have worked on adopting new ways to care for myself each month. I started reading at night when he went to sleep about a month ago. I'm going back to the gym this month. Create space for yourself by working with your partner and other individuals in your life

4. "The days are long, but the years are short," is a bit of advice that has resonated with me. This is a good motto to live by. Your baby may be wailing, they may refuse to nap, the animals may be fighting, and you may be hungry all at once. The moments can be quite difficult. They are difficult. It's difficult to handle everything, no matter how much work you have or how much support you have. But the moment will pass, as will the day, and the days will turn into weeks, and the weeks will turn into years, and before you know it, your child will be the contributing member of society you hoped for.

5. If your anxiety is worsening or you are unable to function, you may have Postpartum Anxiety. Working with a perinatal-trained therapist can be beneficial in your quest to control your symptoms.

Being a new parent and caring for a newborn, infant, toddler, pre-teen, or teen comes with its own set of obstacles that can cause anxiety, worry, and fear at any age. My mother and grandmother still both warn me to be cautious when driving on the highway. Either anxiety runs in families or all mothers are constantly concerned about their children.

Seeking help when needed

Accepting that you may have postpartum depression (PPD) can be difficult. However, communicating the news with your partner, a close family member, a friend, or your doctor can be even more difficult.

While there is a stigma associated with depression and mental health disorders in general, it can be especially difficult to come up about PPD. You may be concerned that these emotions indicate that you aren't cut out to be a mother, or, worse, that you don't truly love your child. (Of course, none of this is real. PPD does not imply that you have something "wrong" with you, and it is not your fault.)

Nevertheless, speaking out is critical. Being open about your feelings can make you feel less alone and is the first step in receiving the treatment you require to feel better.

Why should you disclose that you have PPD?
It may appear that you are in a really dark place right now, with no obvious route out. However, postpartum depression can be treated with talk therapy and/or medication. In fact, seeking treatment is essential for feeling better. Keep in mind that PPD is a serious medical disease. You can't just snap out of it, and it can get worse if you don't receive help.

Telling your partner or someone you trust sets the ball rolling for you to begin receiving that care. Furthermore, your partner or loved one may be able to help you more effectively if they know how you're feeling. (In rare circumstances, it may find out that your partner is experiencing comparable difficulties.)

Once you've informed someone close to you, the next step is to schedule an appointment with your doctor (typically your OB/GYN) as soon as possible so that you can begin receiving the therapy you require immediately.

Talking and getting treated is not only beneficial to your health. It's also the best thing you can do for your baby. PPD can make bonding with your newborn and tending to her needs more difficult.

In a nutshell? You owe it to yourself and your child to recover. And talking about how you're feeling will help you get there.

How to Inform a Partner, Family Member, or Friend about Your PPD

There is no right or wrong way to talk about your depression; what matters is that you feel comfortable doing so. However, structuring the conversation with facts regarding postpartum depression and its symptoms might be an excellent place to start because it sets the stage for discussing your feelings in relation to PPD.

Here's how that may look:

"Can you spare a minute to speak?" I've been researching postpartum depression and its symptoms. Some of these correspond to how I've been feeling, and I'm worried. I'm aware that simply being pregnant and giving birth puts a woman at risk for PPD, and that it's extremely prevalent, impacting up to one in every seven women. "I believe I should discuss my symptoms with my doctor and see if I should seek medical attention.

Of course, if such approach feels too official, you can be more casual. It's quite acceptable to simply ask, "Do you have a minute to talk?" I've been feeling down recently and am concerned that I may be suffering from postpartum depression." When you open up, your companion or loved one will be curious. And from there, you can express your emotions.

How to Inform a Doctor or Medical Professional about Your PPD

At your postpartum appointments, your OB/GYN will likely inquire about PPD symptoms or administer a PPD screening test, and your baby's physician may do the same. If this occurs, strive to give honest answers – don't downplay your feelings. (However, if you are experiencing severe symptoms or are considering killing yourself or your baby, don't wait. Call 911 immediately.)

If your doctor or your baby's physician hasn't specifically asked about PPD, don't be afraid to bring it up. You can simply ask, "Can we talk about postpartum depression?" "I believe I am experiencing some symptoms."

Irrespective of how the discussion begins, when it comes time to share your symptoms, try to be comprehensive and avoid being ashamed. Tell us when they started, how severe they are, and how they affect your daily life. You might say, for example, that about two weeks after giving birth, you started feeling sad for no reason and weren't bonding with your baby, and that sometimes you cry when you can't soothe the baby and have no interest in going for walks, despite the fact that you normally enjoy them.

If your symptoms point to postpartum depression, your doctor or pediatrician can refer you to mental health specialists or other resources that can help you feel better.

More advice on how to ask for help with PPD
The more you express your requirements, the better they will be met. There is no right or wrong way to do it, but these suggestions can help.

•Ask what you need
It could be a few hours of child care so you can s ee a therapist or join a support group, someone t o help with the ever-growing pile of laundry, or t he opportunity to snooze on a Saturday afternoo n.

Those you care about can assist you if you are o
pen about your needs.

•You can inform as many (or as few) individuals as you choose
You don't have to tell everyone you have PPD, but you also don't have to keep it a secret. It is absolutely up to you with whom you discuss your feelings. However, the more trusted people you open up to, the more assistance you may receive. And some family members or acquaintances may respond by saying they have gone through something similar.

•Even if you lack support, seek assistance
Some people are uncomfortable discussing mental health issues. If your partner or family is unwilling to acknowledge your symptoms and the need for treatment, speak with your doctor about receiving help on your own.

•Take someone with you to your doctor's appointment

Having someone with you can help you ensure that you are taking in all of the information the doctor is giving you, especially if it appears to be overwhelming. Your partner or a loved one may be able to provide feedback on your symptoms and how they appear to be impacting you.

•Take part in a support group

PPD support groups can be located at local hospitals, family planning clinics, and community centers. The hospital where you gave birth or your doctor may be able to point you in the right direction.

•Keep in mind that there is nothing "wrong" with you.

PPD is not your fault, and it does not make you insane or a horrible mother. You have a very common and very treatable mental health problem. No new mother is an island, and this is especially true for those who are experiencing post-partum depression. Although discussing your problems with someone else can be difficult, it's the best thing you can do to begin feeling better. Thus, don't delay.

CHAPTER 7

Common Postpartum Body Struggles

Common postpartum body struggles vary from woman to woman, but some experiences are widely shared among new mothers. It's important to note that each woman's body is unique, and the postpartum period is a time of adjustment and recovery.

Addressing physical changes after childbirth

Many changes occur in your body immediately following the birth of a child. Your physique changed dramatically throughout pregnancy. It worked tirelessly to keep your child safe and healthy. Your body is changing again now that your kid is here. Some of these changes are physical, such as your breasts filling up with milk. Others are emotional, such as feeling overly stressed.

Many discomforts and physical changes are usual after giving delivery. However, they are occasionally signs or symptoms of a health problem that requires care. Even if you feel good, it's critical that you attend all of your postpartum visits. These medical checkups allow you to ask your health care physician or health care team questions and can assist your provider in detecting and treating problems.

PHYSICAL CHANGES

1. Perineum discomfort

The perineum is the region between the vagina and the rectum. During labor and vaginal birth, it strains and may tear. It is common to have pain after giving birth, and this may be exacerbated if you have an episiotomy. This is a cut made at the vaginal opening to help your baby come out.

Actions that you can take:

•Perform Kegel exercises. The pelvic muscles get stronger by these activities. Squeeze the muscles that you employ to stop yourself from passing urine (peeing) to perform Kegel exercises. Tighten the muscles for 10 seconds, then relax. Do this at least ten times in a row, three times every day.

•Apply a cold compress on your perineum. Use ice that has been wrapped in a towel. You can also buy cold packs and freeze them in your freezer.

•Place yourself on a pillow or a donut-shaped cushion.

•Take a warm bath.

•Wipe after using the restroom, front to back. As your episiotomy heals, this can help avoid infection.

•Ask your physician about taking painkillers.

2. Afterbirth pains

Stomach cramps, often known as afterbirth symptoms, happen as your uterus (womb) shrinks back to its pre-pregnancy size. The cramping should subside after a few days. Your uterus is round and firm after giving birth and weighs roughly 212 pounds. It weighs only 2 ounces six weeks after birth.

Actions that you can take:

Find out from your doctor what over-the-counter pain relievers are available to you. Medications that you can purchase over-the-counter do not require a prescription from your healthcare professional.

3. Body changes after a c-section

A cesarean delivery, sometimes referred to as a "c-section," is a surgical procedure in which your doctor creates an incision in your abdomen and uterus to deliver your baby. Since a c-section is serious surgery, your recovery period may be prolonged. Because you lost blood during the procedure, you could feel extremely exhausted in the days or weeks following a c-section. Your belly's incision (cut) can hurt.

Actions that you can take:

•Request painkillers from your physician. Consult them before taking any pain relievers.

•Seek assistance from your loved ones, friends, and partner with the infant and around the house.

•When you can, get some sleep. Even if your baby naps during the day, you should still go to bed when they do.

•Avoid lifting while crouching. Nothing heavier than your infant should be lifted.

•When nursing, use pillows to support your growing baby.

•To assist in replenishing the fluids in your body, drink a lot of water.

4. Discharge from the vagina

Your body expels the blood and tissue that were inside your uterus after your baby is born. This is referred to as lochia, or vaginal discharge. It is bright crimson, thick, and may have blood clots in the early days. The flow becomes less and lighter in hue with time. Discharge could last for a few weeks, a month, or longer.

Actions that you can take:

Until the discharge stops, use sanitary pads.

5. Engorgement of the breasts

Your breasts enlarge at this point as they fill with milk. It typically occurs a few days following childbirth. You can have aching and tender breasts. Usually, the soreness subsides as soon as you begin nursing often. It may continue if you're not nursing until your breasts cease producing milk, which normally happens in a few days.

Actions that you can take:

•Breastfeeding is recommended for your infant. Try not to miss a feeding or go too long between them. Night feedings should not be skipped.

•Express a small bit of milk from your breast using a breast pump or by hand before breastfeeding your baby.

•To help your milk flow, take a warm shower or place warm cloths on your breasts. Apply ice packs to your breasts if your engorgement is extremely uncomfortable.

•Wear nursing pads in your bra if your breasts are leaking between feedings to keep your clothes dry.

•Inform your doctor if your breasts remain swollen and uncomfortable.

•Wear a sturdy, supportive bra (such as a sports bra) if you do not intend to breastfeed.

6. Nipple ache

If you're nursing, you may get nipple plainness, especially if your nipples crack.

Actions that you can take:

•Consult your physician or a lactation consultant to ensure that your baby is latching on to your breast correctly. A lactation consultant is someone who has been trained to assist women who are having difficulty nursing. When your baby's mouth is securely attached to (placed around) your nipple, this is referred to as latching on.

•Inquire with your physician about a cream that is safe to use on your nipples to relieve discomfort such as cracking or dryness.

•Rub some breast milk to your nipples after breastfeeding. Allow your breasts to air dry.

7. Swelling

Swelling is common in the hands, feet, and faces of pregnant women. It results from an excess of fluid in your body. After giving birth, it could take some time for the swelling to go down.

Actions that you can take:

•For relaxing or sleeping, lie on your left side.

•Elevate your feet.

•Dress comfortably and try not to overheat.

•Make sure to take a lot of water.

8. Hemorrhoids

Hemorrhoids are uncomfortable, bulging veins that can bleed or ache in the area around the anus. During and after pregnancy, hemorrhoids are frequently experienced.

Actions that you can take:

•Relax in a hot tub.

•Consult your doctor about using a pain reliever that you can buy over-the-counter.

•Take fruits, vegetables, whole-grain breads and cereals, and other high-fiber foods.

•Ensure you take water very well.

•When you're pooping (having a bowel movement), try not to strain.

9. Constipation

Constipation occurs when you do not have bowel motions, have them infrequently, or your stools (poop) are difficult to pass. You may also get unpleasant gas. This may occur for a few days after giving delivery.

Actions that you can take:

•Consume foods high in fiber.

•Taking plenty of water is advised

•Inquire with your doctor about which medications to take.

10. Urinary issues

You may have pain or burning when urinating (peeing) in the first few days after giving birth. You might also try to urinate but find that you can't. You may find it difficult to stop urinating at times. This is known as incontinence. It normally goes away when your pelvic muscles regain strength.

Actions that you can take:

•Consume plenty of water.

•When you go to the bathroom, turn on the water in the sink.

•Take a warm bath.

•Inform your healthcare provider if the discomfort persists.

•Do Kegel exercises to strengthen your pelvic muscles if you have incontinence.

11. Sweating

This is common among new mothers, especially at night. It's caused by your body's altering hormones after pregnancy.

Actions that you can take:

•To keep your sheets and pillow dry, sleep on a towel.

•Wear warm clothes to bed and don't use too many blankets.

12. Tiredness

You could have lost blood during labor and delivery. This can cause exhaustion in your body. And your infant is unlikely to let you sleep through the night!

Actions that you can take:

•Even if your baby naps throughout the day, sleep when your baby sleeps.

•Consume nutritious foods such as fruits and vegetables, whole-grain breads and pasta, and lean meats and poultry. Limit your intake of sweets and high-fat foods.

•Request assistance from your partner, family, and friends with the baby and around the house.

•Visitors should be kept to a bearest minimum. After you've recovered, you'll have plenty of time to present your new baby to family and friends.

13.Worrying about your baby's weight

After giving birth, you lose about 10 pounds right away, and a bit more within the first week. It will take time to shed all of the weight you have acquired. Some women do not immediately shed all of the weight they gained during pregnancy. Most women find this situation very stressful. What matters most is that you eat nutritious foods and engage in physical activity every day. Eating healthy and being physically active every day can help you feel better by increasing your energy level. If you maintain a healthy weight, you are less likely to develop health problems such as diabetes and high blood pressure than if you are overweight (or underweight). And if you get pregnant again or plan to have another baby in the future, it's better to be at a healthy weight before your second pregnancy.

Actions that you can take:

•Have a conversation about your weight with your physician.Consume nutritious foods. Limit your intake of sweets and foods high in unhealthy fat.

•Consume plenty of water.

•Inquire with your doctor about being active, especially if you've had a c-section. Begin to raise your activity level Cautiously and gradually. Walking and swimming are both excellent hobbies for new mothers. Every day, do something active.

•Breastfeed your child. Breastfeeding, which burns calories, can help you lose some of the weight you acquired during pregnancy.

•Do not try to drop a lot of weight so fast. To heal, your body requires nutrients from meals. If you're breastfeeding, losing too much weight too quickly may impair your milk supply.

•Don't beat yourself up if you don't lose weight as rapidly as you'd want. It requires time to get your physique and belly back in shape. It is more vital to stay active and consume nutritious and fresh meals over time than it is to get in shape immediately after giving birth.

14.   Skin Changes

Stretch marks on your tummy may appear where your skin stretched during pregnancy. Some women get them on their thighs, hips, and bottom as well. They do not vanish after giving birth, although they do fade with time.

Actions that you can take:

On your skin, apply creams or lotions. They do not remove stretch marks, but they can help alleviate irritation caused by stretch marks.

15. Hair Changes

During pregnancy, your hair may have appeared thicker and fuller. This is because your body's elevated hormone levels cause you to lose less hair throughout pregnancy. Your hair may begin to thin after the birth of your child. You may possibly get hair loss. Hair loss normally ceases 6 months after giving birth. In a year, your hair should have restored to its typical fullness.

Actions that you can take:

•Consume a lot of fruits and veggies. Your hair may develop and be protected by the nutrients in fruits and vegetables.

•Treat your hair with care. Avoid using tight rollers, braids, or ponytails. These may cause tension and hair pulling.

•Make use of your hair dryer's cool setting.

16. Getting your period again

Six to eight weeks after giving birth, if you're not breastfeeding, your period can start up again. It can take months for it to start up again if you are nursing. Some women don't get their period back until they quit nursing. Your menstrual cycle might not be the same as it was before you were pregnant. It might not be as long as it was. It usually goes back to how it was before you became pregnant over time.

17.Getting pregnant again

In order to give your body time to recuperate after giving birth, many medical professionals advise waiting four to six weeks before having intercourse. When the time comes for sexual activity, use caution as pregnancy might occur before the onset of menstruation. This is because you might not receive your period again until after you ovulate, or release an egg.

Actions that you can take:

Make sure you don't become pregnant again before you're ready by using birth control. Using birth control can help you avoid becoming pregnant. Condoms, implants, the pill, and intrauterine devices—also known as IUDs—are a few forms of birth control. Discuss the best birth control option with your healthcare professional, particularly if you are nursing a baby. Certain birth control methods may cause your milk production to decrease. It is not birth control to breastfeed. Pregnancy is not prevented by it.

It is generally recommended that women wait at least 18 months, or 1.5 years, between pregnancies. Your chance of preterm birth (birth before 37 weeks of pregnancy) increases if you wait too little between pregnancies. Compared to newborns born on schedule, premature babies are more likely to experience health issues. Before it is prepared for your second pregnancy, your body needs time to properly heal from the last one.

CHAPTER 8

Body image issues and societal expectations

Becoming a mother is a wonderful, life-changing experience, but it often comes with many complications, especially when it comes to body image.The false images in the media and on social media platforms, along with societal expectations, might exacerbate body image problems that new mothers may have. Let's examine these difficulties in more detail:

•Get in the "Bounce Back" mood:
Society frequently puts pressure on new moms to get back to their pre-pregnancy figures as soon as possible. Women who are expected to "bounce back" are put under needless stress at a time when they should be recuperating and spending quality time with their newborn.

•Unrealistic Standards and Media Representations:

The media frequently features celebrities who, after having birth, appear to revert to their pre-pregnancy bodies. This inflates expectations and increases feelings of inadequacy in new mothers.

•Culture of Comparison:

Social media's comparison culture has the potential to make problems with body image worse. Self-doubt and unhappiness might result from being exposed to carefully chosen photographs of supposedly ideal postpartum bodies on a regular basis.

•Attention to Outward Appearance:

The amazing physical and emotional journey of parenting can be overshadowed by society's emphasis on outward beauty. Instead of being honored for the incredible achievement of delivering a new life into the world, new moms could feel that their worth is only based on how they look.

•Influence on Mental Well-Being:
The mental health of new mothers can be severely impacted by body image problems, which can lead to tension, anxiety, and even postpartum depression. The happiness of being a first-time mother can sometimes be overshadowed by the pressure from society to fit into a specific body type.

•Cultural Aspects:
The burden placed on new mothers might be exacerbated by cultural norms and expectations. Stress is increased in certain cultures where there is a high emphasis on getting back to pre-pregnancy weight and shape.

•The Change in One's Own Identity:
Self-identity might change as a result of the bodily changes that come with becoming a mother. It can be emotionally taxing to navigate

the difficulties of motherhood while adjusting to a new body image.

Encouraging self-acceptance

It is important for new mothers to embark on a new journey of transformation – a journey of self-acceptance. Here's a heartfelt guide to cultivating self-acceptance as you navigate the beautiful chaos called motherhood.

1. Embrace your postpartum body:
Your body has just accomplished an incredible feat and brought new life into the world. Embrace change, pay attention to its signs, and be grateful for the strength that allowed you to hold your little one in your arms.

2. Celebrate milestones big and small:
Celebrate small wins, from nutritious meals to a little self-care. Every success, no matter how small it may seem, is a step forward in your journey to motherhood.

3. Practice self-compassion:

Treat yourself with the same kindness and understanding you would show your child. Know that you are in uncharted territory and it's okay to not have all the answers.

4. Shift your focus from "backwards" to "forwards."

Instead of fixating on getting back to your pre-pregnancy state, focus on moving forward. Your body is on a journey and every step is progress. It's not about recovery. It is about promoting the body's resilience and development.

5. Surround yourself with positivity:

Build a support system that encourages and encourages you. Surround yourself with people who appreciate your journey and celebrate your own evolving beauty.

6. Find joy in the moments of motherhood:

Even in the diaper changes and sleepless nights, find joy in the simple moments of motherhood.

Appreciate your baby's giggles, your pinky wrapped around your baby's fingers, and the warmth of your embrace. These moments are the true treasures of motherhood.

7. Set realistic expectations:

Let go of unrealistic expectations from both society and yourself and understand that there is no one-size-fits-all approach to motherhood. Your journey is unique and embracing chaos and imperfection is a beautiful thing.

8. Prioritize self-care:

Plan some time for self-care, even if it's only for a short time. Cherish the moments that recharge your mind, whether it's a hot cup of tea, a quick walk, or a few minutes of quiet reflection.

9. Think about your strengths:

Take a moment to think about the strengths that have supported you as a mother along the way. Recognize your resilience, adaptability, and love as the driving force behind your journey.

10. Seek professional help if necessary:
If you're still feeling unsure or overwhelmed, don't hesitate to seek professional help. A psychologist or support group can provide guidance and a safe space to express your feelings.

Remember that being a new mom is not about perfection, it's about growing, learning, and being open-minded and embracing the journey. You are enough just the way you are. Through self-acceptance, you not only nurture yourself, but you also create a foundation of love and acceptance for the precious life you are now nurturing. Accept the special woman you have become and keep growing.

CHAPTER 9

Antidepressants in Postpartum Depression

Meaning of Antidepressants

Antidepressants are drugs for treatment of depression. They have neurotransmitter effects, lower the biological impact of stress on the brain, reduce neuroinflammation - inflammation in the brain or spinal cord - and boost the brain's capacity to deal with future stress.

They do not work instantly; you may feel the effects after a few weeks. There are various types of antidepressants, and you may need to try several before finding the one that works best for you.

Research on PPD has mostly focused on medications currently used to treat anxiety and depression, such as antidepressants. Nevertheless, the FDA has not expressly approved these drugs to treat the illness. While there is one drug specifically licensed for PPD, Zulresso, most treatments are administered off-label.

The best first treatment for mild to moderate PPD is typically psychotherapy. However, medicine can also be beneficial for a lot of people. In this section,a few particular drugs that your doctor might recommend if you are found to have PPD will be discussed.

1.Selective serotonin reuptake inhibitors(SSRIs)
The FDA has licensed selective serotonin reuptake inhibitors (SSRIs) for a number of illnesses, including anxiety and depression. Off-label, they are also used to treat PPD.

They generally function by altering serotonin, a neurotransmitter that may be involved in mood. For PPD, there are no SSRIs with FDA approval. However, some SSRIs, such as sertraline (Zoloft), fluoxetine (Prozac), and paroxetine (Paxil), have been examined for the treatment of PPD.

In a 2013 research, the sertraline group experienced considerably higher rates of response and remission—a time during which there are no symptoms of depression—than the placebo group (a pill that contains no medication).

The advantages of taking an SSRI typically exceed the disadvantages if you are nursing. Due to its lower tendency to enter breast milk, sertraline is a frequently given medication. However, before taking any medication, make sure your healthcare professional is aware that you are nursing. We have an article on SSRIs, breastfeeding, and pregnancy that has additional information on this subject.

Additionally, don't forget to inform your provider if you've previously experienced success with an SSRI treatment for depression. Given that it has previously worked for you, they might want to start there.

It could take up to four weeks after starting an SSRI before you start to feel better. You'll probably need to keep taking it for six months to a year if it succeeds. Your doctor could advise gradually reducing your dosage and eventually quitting the medicine if you continue to have symptoms after that.

SSRIs are often well-tolerated drugs with few persistent adverse effects. The largest exclusions are adverse effects related to sex, which are more likely to persist if they do.

2. SNRIs (serotonin-norepinephrine reuptake inhibitors)

Another type of antidepressant that is frequently used off-label to treat PPD is serotonin-norepinephrine reuptake inhibitors (SNRIs). They primarily function by increasing serotonin and norepinephrine, two brain chemicals.

An example of an SNRI used to treat PPD is venlafaxine (Effexor). A tiny 2001 trial on venlafaxine for PPD indicated that after 8 weeks of treatment, 12 of the 15 individuals obtained PPD remission. SNRIs may be useful, but they're normally only taken if SSRIs aren't working or if you've previously had success with an SNRI.

Although data is sparse, there is indication that venlafaxine may be a viable option during nursing. Again, before taking any medicine while nursing, always consult with your healthcare professional. The adverse effects of SNRIs are similar to those of SSRIs, except they can induce more nausea, sleeping issues, dry mouth, and blood pressure fluctuations. Like SSRIs, most side effects fade over time.

3. Wellbutin(Bupropion)

Bupropion is an antidepressant that has been licensed by the FDA for the treatment of severe depression and seasonal affective disorder (SAD). It increases the levels of particular brain chemicals (norepinephrine and dopamine) that are thought to influence mood. However, researchers do not fully comprehend how this works.

A short 2005 research on bupropion for PPD found that it significantly improved depressed symptoms. However, the researchers noted that sertraline or venlafaxine medication increased the likelihood of PPD remission.

Bupropion may potentially be utilized as a therapeutic option during nursing, but research on this is limited.. As previously said, if you are nursing, speak with your healthcare professional about your alternatives. Bupropion has similar side effects to SSRIs and SNRIs, however it is less likely to induce sexual issues.

4. Nortriptyline

Nortriptyline, a tricyclic antidepressant (TCA), is extensively used to treat depression. Nortriptyline is hypothesized to work on a variety of chemical messengers in the central nervous system, with norepinephrine and serotonin being its primary targets.

A 2006 trial on nortriptyline treatment for PPD found that it improved depressive symptoms similarly to sertraline. There is some evidence that it may be as effective as SSRIs or psychotherapy for PPD. TCAs, on the other hand, have more adverse effects than SSRIs, such as dry mouth, impaired vision, and sleepiness. As a result, they aren't usually the first-line treatment for depression.

5. Zulresso

Zulresso (brexanolone) was approved by the FDA in 2019. It is the first and only FDA-approved treatment for PPD.

It could be an option for you if you:
•PPD has been diagnosed in you.

•You must be at least 15 years old.
•You do not have severe renal disease.

Zulresso is a synthetic form of allopregnanolone, a hormone-related chemical produced by the body from progesterone. When you're pregnant, your body produces a lot of allopregnanolone. However, allopregnanolone levels drop dramatically after giving birth. Zulresso replenishes the supplies in your body.

Although researchers are not so sure how Zulresso works, it seems to help with depression. It's probable that it affects your brain's GABA system, which is involved in mood regulation.

In various respects, Zulresso differs from the antidepressants listed above. Here's what you should know:

•It's not a pill, but rather an infusion. Zulresso is not something you take at home. It is administered via IV (intravenous) infusion over a 2.5-day period. This implies that after receiving the infusion, you must stay overnight in a specific treatment center for many days.

•It only takes three days to complete.Zulresso has been shown to help some people feel better in 3 days or less. Antidepressants (such as those described above) take 1 to 2 months to fully kick in.

•There may be obstacles to receiving therapy. Zulresso costs more than $30,000. Zulresso is sometimes covered by health insurance, but only if you satisfy certain criteria (such as first attempting an oral antidepressant or delivering birth within the previous 6 months). Zulresso's manufacturer also offers many financial aid programs to help you pay for the drug.

•You must be watched 24 hours a day. Zulresso can sedate you and possibly cause you to pass out. As a result, you must be monitored by a healthcare provider 24 hours a day during the infusion. Dry mouth and flushing of the skin or face are also common adverse effects.

•Zulresso was compared to placebo in a 2018 trial that included two investigations and approximately 200 participants with PPD. Zulresso was more effective than placebo in treating PPD in these studies. The data was strong enough for the FDA to designate Zulresso as a breakthrough therapy and promptly authorize it for usage. This suggests that the FDA believes Zulresso is as successful as, if not better than, any other PPD medication now available.

Insight into the role of antidepressants in treatment

Antidepressants serve an important role in the treatment of postpartum depression (PPD), providing relief to moms facing emotional difficulties following childbirth. However, it is critical to emphasize that the choice to utilize antidepressants to treat postpartum depression should be decided cooperatively by the mother and her healthcare professional. Each woman's condition is unique, and a personalized strategy that takes into account the intensity of symptoms, individual preferences, and potential side effects is critical for the best possible results. Antidepressants roles includes:

Balancing Neurotransmitters:
Antidepressants, particularly selective serotonin reuptake inhibitors (SSRIs) and serotonin-norepinephrine reuptake inhibitors (SNRIs), work by increasing the levels of neurotransmitters such as serotonin and norepinephrine in the brain. These neurotransmitters play an important role in mood regulation.

Alleviating Depressive Symptoms:
Postpartum depression often involves a range of symptoms, including persistent sadness, anxiety, and irritability. Antidepressants are effective in alleviating these symptoms, allowing mothers to experience more stable and positive emotions.

Managing Hormonal Changes:

Significant hormonal variations, particularly a rapid drop in estrogen and progesterone levels, characterize the postpartum period. Antidepressants can help reduce the negative effects of hormonal fluctuations on mood and emotional well-being.

Improving Sleep Habits:
Sleep problems are frequent in postpartum depression and can exacerbate symptoms. Antidepressants may assist improve sleep patterns by regulating mood, giving new moms much-needed rest.

Increasing Therapy Effectiveness:
Antidepressants are frequently used in conjunction with psychotherapy to improve the efficacy of therapeutic therapies. When medicine is used with counseling or cognitive-behavioral therapy, it is possible to address both the medical and psychological elements of postpartum depression.

Reducing the Chances of Relapse:

Antidepressants can lower the chance of relapse in people who have previously experienced depression. Maintaining medication may give continued protection against relapse for mothers who have experienced depression prior to pregnancy or throughout past postpartum periods.

Making Daily Functioning Possible:
Antidepressants assist moms to participate more completely in their daily lives by reducing depression symptoms, such as caring for their newborns, maintaining relationships, and participating in social events. This adds to a general improvement in life quality.

Breastfeeding Mothers' Support:
Some antidepressants are deemed breastfeeding friendly, allowing moms to continue nursing while undergoing therapy. Healthcare experts can assist women in selecting drugs that provide the fewest hazards to the infant while breastfeeding.

Increasing Emotional Stability:

Antidepressants promote emotional stability by lowering the severity of mood swings and allowing mothers to react to the demands of parenting with greater resilience.

Creating a Pathway to Recovery:

Antidepressants can provide a temporary bridge to recovery for some mothers. As therapy, support, and lifestyle changes take effect, some people may be able to go off medication with the help of their healthcare practitioners.

CHAPTER 10

Clear information on potential benefits and risks of antidepressants

The Benefits of Antidepressants

Taking antidepressants has numerous advantages. Being aware of these advantages can assist you in making an informed decision.

•They are excellent for symptom relief

Antidepressants have been shown to be more successful than placebo in treating serious depression in adults, though they often take a few weeks to take effect, and you may need to try more than one to discover the best effective antidepressant for you.

•They have been thoroughly researched and are generally considered safe

The Food and Drug Administration (FDA) has authorized all antidepressants. This means they have undergone extensive testing and clinical trials.

•They can assist you in completing other aspects of your treatment plan

Your treatment plan may include a variety of activities, such as doing basic self-care tasks. If you are apathetic and lethargic as a result of your depression, antidepressants can help restore your energy so you can complete everyday tasks, participate in therapy, and other items on your treatment plan.

•Improved living quality

People who use antidepressants report an enhanced quality of life in addition to mood advantages.They are less reactive to bad life experiences, can examine things in a more balanced manner, and can concentrate better.

Antidepressants' potential drawbacks

Antidepressants, like any drug, can have drawbacks. These may vary from person to person, but being aware of them can help you prepare. Speaking with your doctor about any of the disadvantages can help you reevaluate your prescription. The negatives must be weighed against the benefits in this discussion.

•You may need to try a few before you spot the appropriate one for you.

Not every antidepressant will be suitable for everyone. You may need to alter medications more than once to discover the optimum one for you and your symptoms.

•They may have an impact on your sexual drive.

Antidepressants may impair sexual desire or function. Some antidepressants are more prone to cause sexual adverse effects than others. One in every five adults in the United States develops sexual side effects as a result of antidepressants. This can involve delayed lubrication, orgasm that is delayed or obstructed, or difficulty sustaining an erection. If the side effects are interfering with your relationship, talk to your doctor about reducing the dosage or finding other ways to deal with them.

•They may have an impact on your sleep and/or weight.

Although insomnia is a typical complaint among persons suffering from depression, it is not always obvious if it is a side effect of medicine or a lingering symptom of depression. In the end, antidepressants may help to normalize sleep over time. However, depending on the antidepressant, the dosage, and the time of day you take it, certain antidepressants may lead to insomnia, while others may be overly sedating. If you have a sleep issue, this can exacerbate your sleep problems. Consult your doctor if your antidepressant is interfering with your sleep. The medication or dosage may need to be reconsidered.

Weight gain is an adverse effect of several antidepressants. Everyone is unique and reacts differently to drugs. Weight gain can occur when regular activities such as meal preparation or socializing with friends resume and entail eating. An enhanced mood might also increase your appetite. Other antidepressants are less likely to cause weight gain. Overall, the risk of weight gain should not be considered while choosing an antidepressant.

•They could be expensive.
Even with insurance and generic prescriptions, some patients may find the drug prohibitively expensive. Although prescription costs are determined by your insurance provider and plan, it may be beneficial to work with your doctor to determine whether the doctor needs to submit an authorization request to your insurance company, assist you in finding a more affordable option, or provide you with samples or coupons.

•They may have unintended consequences.

Side symptoms such as dry mouth, weariness, nausea, or headache might be bothersome, especially at initially. The good news is that these small side effects usually fade away within a few weeks. Consult your doctor if you continue to have adverse effects or if other major negative effects persist.

•You cannot stop abruptly if you choose to stop.

If you decide to discontinue taking antidepressants, do so gradually as withdrawal symptoms can arise. Do not discontinue your medicine until you have spoken with your doctor. They may put you on a tapering schedule or move you to a different drug. They can also keep an eye out for withdrawal symptoms.

In general, antidepressants are a safe and effective therapy choice for depression. There are many antidepressant classes and medications within each class. Finding the correct one for you can take some time, and you may have to test several before you find the one that works best for you.

Can talk therapy be an option for treatment of PPD?

Yes! Therapy is an excellent alternative for treating PPD, especially if your symptoms are mild or moderate. Therapy works equally as effectively as medication for many people. Among the options are:

Cognitive behavioral therapy (CBT): CBT entails discussing your thoughts, actions, and feelings with a counselor or therapist. It is a first-line treatment for PPD, either alone or in conjunction with medication. One can actually used CBT for a few months. In some circumstances, even a one-day workshop can be beneficial.

Interpersonal therapy is concerned with how your connections, obligations, and life experiences influence your mood. It is a first-line treatment for PPD, just like CBT.

Other treatments: PPD can be helped by a variety of various sorts of therapy. Non-directive counseling, peer counseling, behavioral activation treatment, and psychodynamic psychotherapy are examples.

Remember that therapy can take place in person or via the internet (telehealth). There are other smartphone apps that provide therapy. Joining a peer support group is another excellent approach to connect with others who are going through similar experiences.

Special focus on effects for breastfeeding mothers and infants

The effects of antidepressants on breastfeeding mothers and infants may vary depending on the drug used, the dose, and individual factors. It is important for breastfeeding mothers to discuss the potential risks and benefits with their health care provider to make an informed decision. Generally, here are some considerations.

1. Transfer of drugs into breast milk:
Most antidepressants pass into breast milk, but in varying amounts. Some drugs have low concentrations in breast milk, minimizing exposure to the infant.

2. Selective serotonin reuptake inhibitors (SSRIs) and serotonin norepinephrine reuptake inhibitors (SNRIs):
SSRIs and SNRIs are commonly prescribed antidepressants. These drugs are considered safe during breastfeeding, but reactions may vary from person to person. It is important to monitor the infant for possible side effects.

3. Possible side effects in infants:
Most infants exposed to antidepressants through breast milk do not experience side effects. However, possible side effects include restlessness, sleep disturbances, and changes in eating habits. These side effects are often moderate and temporary.

4. Individual drug profile:

Different antidepressants have different profiles for their passage into breast milk. Some have been more extensively studied and are considered safer options during breastfeeding.

5. Timing of medication:

Taking the drug immediately after breastfeeding can minimize the concentration of the drug in breast milk during the next feeding. It is important to discuss the best timing with your healthcare provider.

6. Close monitoring by healthcare providers:

Health care providers closely monitor breastfeeding mothers and infants when antidepressants are prescribed. Regular examinations allow us to assess the health of mother and child and quickly address possible side effects.

7. Weigh risks and benefits:

Taking antidepressants while breastfeeding requires careful consideration of the risks and benefits. For some mothers, the benefits of treating postpartum depression may outweigh the risks of drug exposure.

8. Individualized treatment plan:

Treatment plans are highly individualized and take into account the specific needs and circumstances of each mother-infant pair. Health care providers will consider the severity of the mother's symptoms, the potential impact on breastfeeding, and the overall health of both parties.

9. Consultation with a lactation specialist:

In some cases, consulting a breastfeeding specialist may provide additional guidance about breastfeeding while taking antidepressants. A lactation specialist can provide insight to maintain your milk supply and manage breastfeeding issues.

10. Alternative treatment options:

If the risks associated with antidepressants are a concern, alternative treatment options such as psychotherapy, support groups, and lifestyle interventions may be considered. These alternatives may be effective for some people.

Women who are breastfeeding should be honest with their health care provider about their concerns and wishes. Together, they can make informed decisions that prioritize both the mother's mental health and the infant's well-being. Regular monitoring and changing the treatment plan as needed contributes to a safe and supportive environment for mother and child.

CHAPTER 11

Practical Tips for the Fourth Trimester

Everyone talks about the three trimesters of pregnancy, the changes in your body, and how your kid grows in the womb, which makes sense.

After all, pregnancy is a significant event, and monitoring your and your baby's health is critical!

However, as much as pregnancy might turn your life upside down, having your baby in your arms may be an even more momentous adjustment. It's a big change for you, and it should be treated as seriously as your first three trimesters of pregnancy.

The fourth trimester refers to the first few months of postpartum parenthood. You and your kid are both adjusting to new conditions.

Your kid must adjust to life outside of the safe confines of the womb. And you must allow your body to heal, deal with sleep deprivation, and adjust to being a parent to a newborn.

As difficult as it can be, your fourth trimester can also be a period of joy and good health. Remember, no one is a perfect parent from the start! Laugh, give yourself lots of grace, and follow these self-care practices.

Tips for surviving the fourth trimester

1) Make a Strategy

Whether you're still pregnant or have already given birth, now is the time to prepare a game plan! Consider methods you may practice self-care in advance, and make a list of specific persons who are willing to assist you. To get you started, here are a few examples:

•Make a list of folks who are willing to cook or go grocery shopping with you.

•Purchase postpartum necessities include as pads, witch hazel pads, and nursing pads.

•Make a generic grocery list to provide to others who offer to handle your shopping.

•Make a list of who is available to help with the infant or pick up your older children from school.

•Schedule house cleaning services in advance.

•Schedule time for both you and your partner to engage in pleasurable, uncomplicated self-care activities.

2) Assign Specific Tasks to Friends

When friends and relatives say, "Let me know how I can help," you should take them up on their offer!

Don't always wait for them to suggest a way to help. Your loved ones want to help, but they may be unaware of the exact tasks you require assistance with. So notify them!

Provide tangible strategies for friends and family to help you.

Offer specific methods for friends and family to help you by stating, "Hey, it would be really helpful if you could come over and do my laundry," or "Do you have time to swing by the store and pick up some groceries?"

If you have other children, ask if they could take them to a park for a special playdate or out for an ice cream cone. Siblings may feel left out when a new baby joins the family, so having someone spend focused time with them can be really beneficial.

3) Put your mind at ease
Part of what makes the fourth trimester difficult is that you may be concerned about your baby's safety.

When your child goes down for a nap or to bed at night, your worry can increase significantly, especially if they sleep in their own room. It's natural to be concerned when you can't see your baby!

Take a deep breath and do everything you can to relax your mind. Following safe sleep principles will allow you to rest assured that your kid is resting as safely as possible!

These guidelines are as follows:
•Using a firm cot mattress that is properly fitted for your baby
•Taking out crib cushions, crib bumpers, blankets, and toys
•A bedside sleeper will share your room but not your bed.
•Sleeping your child on their back
•Putting your kid to bed with a pacifier

You should also put your baby to sleep on a breathable mattress, such as Newton Baby's Crib Mattress. That way, if your child rolls over in the middle of the night, you'll know they'll be able to breathe through the mattress!

4) Take a nap

Your baby isn't the only one who should sleep! Sleeping through the night may not be possible for the first few weeks with your infant. Make up for it by getting some shut-eye throughout the day when your baby sleeps.

While it's tempting to utilize this time to catch up on housework or tackle the never-ending laundry pile, doing so is a bad idea in the beginning. You require sleep more than you require a spotless home. Even if you can't sleep, placing your feet up on the couch will provide your body with much-needed rest.

So put the broom down and step away from the washing and dryer. Instead, head to your bed or another comfortable area where you may rest for a time.

Try these tips if you're having problems sleeping during the day:
•Install blackout curtains to make the room darker.

•Let your phone be in another room.

•Listen to music or a radio broadcast to enjoy background noise without being exposed to blue light.

•Lower your intake of caffeine

•Maintain a temperature of 65 degrees in your room.

If there's an issue, ask your partner or a friend to wake you up - knowing someone else is in charge can sometimes help your thoughts relax enough to fall asleep.

5) Consult Your Doctor

If you're still pregnant, talk to your doctor about the 4th trimester now: what services are available, when your postpartum appointment will be, if any medications will need to be adjusted during that time, and what to expect in the weeks following your baby's delivery.

You should also inquire about red flags that signal a concern. Postpartum hypertension, for example, can cause you to see spots or sparkles.

A strong headache is also possible. Infections might also be indicated by a high temperature or red streaks. Knowing the warning signs can help you obtain the medical attention you require.

Furthermore, if you are already in your fourth trimester, you should consult with your doctor about how you're doing, especially if you're having trouble getting rid of the baby blues.

Most women see a postpartum doctor six weeks after giving birth. However, if you have any concerns before this visit, please contact your doctor.

6) Keep an eye out for signs of postpartum depression

PPD is more than just a few miserable days after giving birth. It's a dangerous mental illness that strikes one in every seven women after giving birth and can lead to long-term problems if left untreated. Constant anxiety, eating more or less than normal, disinterest in your infant, family, and friends, and sudden or inexplicable rage are all warning indicators. The majority of these indications are discussed in this book's first chapter. Call your doctor again if you have any questions or are confused.

7) Eat well and move your body

The body is connected to the mind and vice versa. Proper diet and exercise not only help your body stay healthy and heal, but also help you maintain the right mood.

When it comes to physical activity, start with short, easy exercises and be sure to ask your doctor what physical activity you are allowed to do after giving birth (especially important if you had a Caesarean section).

But even if you want to start moving again, there's no need to rush into anything. Stretching too quickly can lead to pelvic pain, urinary leakage, and other problems. Slow down and be attentive to your body. If there is heavy bleeding again, it is a sign that you have overdone it.

8) Help your baby adjust

Remember that your newborn is also going through major changes. You and your baby are together, so do everything you can to help your baby adjust to life outside the womb.

Hold her tightly, bounce and rock her to ensure plenty of skin-to-skin contact, and wrap her comfortably in her swaddle.

Choose a breathable blanket made from 100% organic muslin cotton to keep your lover safe, comfortable, and cozy. Once you've found your favorite blanket, here are some tips. Keep a few of these swaddle blankets on hand. Can also be used as a stroller cover, blanket, burp cloth, or nursing cover.

9) Attempt skin-to-skin contact

You and your baby can benefit from skin-to-skin contact. So, remove the baby's diaper and place it on your bare chest. Then cover your back with a light blanket and snuggle together in bed.

Spending skin-to-skin time will strengthen the bond between you and your newborn.

There are other benefits, including for your baby:
•regulate body temperature
•Increased oxygen levels in the blood
•improve brain development
•developing a strong immune system
•less cry

It also offers a variety of benefits for you, including:
•make more milk
•Lower your risk of postpartum depression
•reduce postpartum bleeding
•Focus on rest to recover
•It's a simple exercise with many rewards. Give your baby skin-to-skin time if needed.

10) Always stay hydrated

Drinking adequate water is always important, but especially during your fourth trimester. This will not only help you heal faster, but it will also ensure that you can produce the milk your baby requires if you are nursing.

11) Consume Enough Food

Your body has just been put through the ringer and requires some fuel. The fourth trimester is not the time for rigorous diets or calorie counting.

If you're hungry, it's for a good cause. Consume a variety of nutritious foods. Here are some strategies for dealing with hunger throughout the fourth trimester:

•Instead of three huge meals, eat numerous smaller ones.

•Keep healthful food in easily accessible places (more on this below!)

•Consume plenty of fruits and veggies to keep your system moving (you don't want to deal with constipation on top of everything else).

To increase milk production, try incorporating oats and other whole grains.

•Avoid excessive sugar consumption.

•Keep track of any meals that seem to bother your child (you may need to change your diet if they develop allergies or food sensitivities).

•Consume protein with each meal to aid in recovery.

•Pay attention to your body. There could be a reason behind your cravings.

•While feeling hungry after childbirth is common, not every new mother will. Some people have little or no appetite. If that describes you, you'll need to make every bite count.

12) Choose Your Snacks Wisely

Snacks can be quite beneficial to your 4th-trimester recovery. They can provide an energy boost to help you keep going when you're feeling tired. Snacks allow you to ingest additional nutrients as well.

However, just because you're hungry doesn't mean you have to eat an entire bag of cookies or chips. Instead, you must choose your snacks wisely.

To achieve that goal, follow these suggestions:
•Keep snacks next to where you feed your infant (so you can easily reach them).
•Keep a variety of foods on hand so you have options.
•Choose easy-to-eat pre-packaged snacks.
•Keep baby wipes or a towel available; you're bound to drop a few crumbs on your baby's head.

Don't be concerned if you're unsure what to eat. Here are some suggestions:
Granola bars
Cookies for lactation
Mandarin oranges or other fruits
Almonds and dried fruit
Sticks of cheese
Eggs that have been hard-boiled
Trail mix
Kefir or yogurt
Popcorn
Hummus and cucumber slices
Carrots and peanut butter

Ants on a log (celery with peanut butter and raisins)
Muffins
Jerky
Energy balls
Slices of bell pepper
Toast with cheese
Dark chocolate

13) Be Ready for Strange Symptoms

While there is a lot of information available online concerning pregnancy symptoms, not as many people discuss what can happen to your body after childbirth. Here are a few examples of what you might encounter:

•Hair loss (particularly if you had magnificent, full locks during pregnancy)
•Hormonal acne breakouts
•If you're breastfeeding, you may get sore, cracked nipples.
•Eyes that are bloodshot
•Aches all across your body as your ligaments re-adjust

•If you have a C-section, you may experience numbness around your scar.

•Hot flashes or chills

•Odd-smelling discharge – but consult your doctor if it's particularly unpleasant.

•Severe gas pain that mimics phantom baby kicks

•Crying over seemingly insignificant matters

If you have any concerns about something you're experiencing, consult your doctor for advice.

14) Keep Your Mind Active

When you're recovering after delivery, one of the worst things you can do is sit and think about everything that could go wrong. If you let it, your imagination can run wild, especially when dealing with hormonal fluctuations.

Find strategies to keep your brain active to assist prevent this from happening. You could try:

•Examine a book or a magazine

•Listen to an audiobook or podcast.

•Perform a word search or a crossword puzzle.

•Fill in the blanks in the baby book.

•Create a tale about your birth.

•Pick up a new skill, such as knitting or scrapbooking.

•Meditate

These focused chores might also help you maintain your mental sharpness. This is especially useful if you have "mom brain" or are feeling a little foggy-headed.

15) Accept Survival Mode

No matter how many children you've had, the fourth trimester is always difficult. Recognize that you will go into survival mode for a while. And be okay with it.

You want to keep things as basic as possible during this period. You may:

•Use disposable plates and cups.

•Keep your meals basic.

•Allow the majority of the housework to pile up.

•Watch more television than normal

•Make rest and mental wellness a priority.
•Snuggle your child
•Remind yourself that this phase will not last forever.

16) Communicate With Your Partner

Everyone in the family changes their lives when they have a baby. Regardless of the changes, your lover is not a mind reader.

That is why you must express your wants and desires clearly. If you require assistance, request it. Teach your partner what it means to be helpful during this difficult time. Because they're probably a little lost and could use some direction.

If they're confused what to do, these Postpartum advice can help. Send this resource to your spouse for review because it has multiple practical instances of showing up for your partner after childbirth.

17) Recognize that it does not last forever.

Your world appears to be turned upside down right now. Everything is different. And you're having trouble making sense of it all.

The good news is that you will eventually find your new normal. Things will be less chaotic by the time your baby is two or three months old. You'll feel more at ease as a mother. And your body will be on its path to healing.

So, if you're in the trenches in the beginning, remember that you won't be there forever.
Life will never be the same again once you give birth, yet better days are ahead of you. This will pass.

Balancing self-care and baby care

Balancing self-care with baby care is an important element of new mothers' overall well-being. Here are some helpful hints for striking a balance between taking care of yourself and caring for your baby:

1. Make self-care a priority:

Schedule Self-Care Time: Make time for self-care activities, such as a short nap, a bath, or time to pursue a hobby. Self-care should be a non-negotiable aspect of your daily routine.

2. Include Your Child in Self-Care:

Combine Activities: Consider incorporating your infant into your self-care routine. Take a soothing bath with your baby, do moderate yoga with your infant nearby, or go for a leisurely stroll with the stroller.

3. Sleep When Your Baby Sleeps:

Prioritize sleep: Sleep is essential for both you and your kid. Consider taking a nap yourself when your baby is sleeping. Avoid the temptation to spend this time for housework and instead prioritize your own health.

4. Assign Tasks:

Delegate work: If possible, delegate work to partners, family members, or friends. Sharing responsibilities helps you to have uninterrupted moments of self-care.

5. Establish a Support System:

Create a Support System: Surround yourself with people who understand the value of self-care. Having someone on whom you can rely for assistance can make it easier to find time for oneself.

6. Establish Realistic Expectations:

Accept Imperfection: Recognize that you will not be able to achieve everything flawlessly. Set realistic goals for yourself and be gentle with yourself if things don't go as planned.

7. Choose Your Baby Gear Wisely:

Invest in Practical Equipment: Use infant equipment that allows you to multitask. A baby carrier or sling, for example, can free up your hands while keeping your baby close, allowing you to engage in self-care activities.

8. Combining Baby Care with Exercise:

Include Your Baby in fitness: Include your baby in your fitness program by engaging in activities that involve your baby. This could involve postpartum workouts or stroller walks through the park.

9. Accept Assistance:

take Help kindly: If someone offers to help, take it kindly. Whether it's a family member making a dinner or a friend keeping the infant, accepting help helps you to prioritize your health.

10. Establish Boundaries:

Communicate Your Needs: Inform those around you about your self-care requirements. Setting clear boundaries helps others understand how important your well-being is to you.

11. Arrange for Outings:

Plan Social Outings: Plan social outings with your infant to socialize and get away from the norm. Meeting other parents or friends might be a novel approach to incorporate self-care into your routine.

12. Meal Planning:

Optimize Meal Planning: Plan and prepare nutritious meals ahead of time to ensure you have enough energy. Consider batch cooking or asking friends or family for dinner assistance.

13. Pay Attention to Your Body:

Prioritize Your Health: Pay attention to the cues sent by your body. Take it if you need it. Eat, if you're hungry. Putting your health first benefits both you and your child.

Balancing self-care and baby care is a constant effort that necessitates adaptability and flexibility. You can build a more harmonious schedule that supports your physical, emotional, and mental well-being throughout the postpartum time by integrating these ideas.

CHAPTER 12

Time-management strategies for new moms

3 Time Management Strategies for Moms

Time is often perceived as a scarce resource when managing a home, raising children, and juggling a career. That is why time management strategies are essential for mothers. Here are some essential strategies for making the most of your day.

1. Organize and Prioritize Your Daily Tasks

The first step is to prioritize tasks. It is not about cramming more tasks into your day; rather, it is about focusing on what is truly important. You should determine the importance and urgency of tasks. Give priority to tasks that are both urgent and important. Tasks that are less urgent but still important can be scheduled for later. Are there any tasks that are neither urgent nor important? Consider whether they are truly necessary.

You can follow this simple table for prioritization:

Priority Urgency Importance
High   High   High
Medium Low   High
Low   Low   Low

This strategy can assist you in organizing your day and ensuring that the most important tasks are not overlooked.

2. Create a Routine

Next, consider developing a routine. A consistent routine can provide structure and predictability to your day by acting as a framework. It's not about sticking to a strict schedule; rather, it's about creating a flow that fits your lifestyle and commitments.

Morning routines can help you start the day off right, while evening routines can help you wind down and prepare for a good night's sleep. Remember that your routine should serve you, not the other way round. It should be adaptable enough to change as your needs change and flexible enough to accommodate unexpected events.

3. Establish Realistic Goals

Finally, set attainable objectives. Setting overly ambitious goals for the day and then feeling frustrated when they are not met is an easy trap to fall into. Remember that you are a mother, not a superhero. Setting realistic goals can increase your productivity and sense of accomplishment.

Break larger tasks down into smaller, more manageable ones. This can help you track your progress throughout the day and make your to-do list seem less daunting. Plus, there's something incredibly satisfying about crossing tasks off your list one by one!

Practical Time Management Tricks for Moms

A few doable tactics can go a long way toward helping you become an expert in the art of time management. Let's look at some essential time management techniques and advice for mothers that will help you make the most of your day.

1. Employ Time-Management Tools

You have access to a wide range of time management tools in the digital age. These tools, which range from task management apps to digital calendars, can assist you in maintaining organization, setting priorities, and monitoring your schedule. Digital calendars can be used to plan out time for particular tasks, set reminders, and schedule appointments. On the other hand, task management applications let you make to-do lists, assign tasks to others, and even set deadlines.

For instance, you can use Magical to automate your repetitive messages, have it draft your emails, and have it fill out forms for kids.

2. Assigning Tasks

Knowing how to assign work is another essential component of efficient time management. It's simple for mothers to get caught up in the trap of trying to handle everything on their own. On the other hand, assigning chores to others can help you focus on the things that really need your full attention, free up time, and lower stress.

Older children, for example, can take on certain responsibilities, such as cleaning their rooms or assisting with meal preparation. If you're working, don't be afraid to delegate tasks to your coworkers in order to better manage your workload. More information on delegation can be found in our article on tips for first-time managers.

3. When it's required, say "No"

Finally, don't be afraid to say no when appropriate. It is critical to understand that you cannot do everything and be everywhere at the same time. Saying no to tasks or commitments that do not align with your priorities or that you simply do not have time for is an essential component of effective time management.

Remember that saying no does not imply that you are failing or not doing enough. It means you're making deliberate choices about how to spend your time.

These practical suggestions can have a big impact on how you manage your time as a mom. You can create a more balanced and manageable schedule by using time management tools, delegating tasks, and learning to say no.

CONCLUSION

As we near the end of our journey through the complex web of new motherhood, it's important to reflect on the real challenges and triumphs that shape these changing times. The stories of biological mothers reflect shared experiences, worries, and joys, forming a unique narrative for each woman who enters the realm of parenting.

In the maze of sleepless nights, soothing lullabies, and diaper changes, self-care can feel like a distant dream. But as the story progresses, similar threads emerge. That is the importance of employing practical leadership that recognizes the complexity of this amazing journey. Three mothers share their experiences with postpartum depression, how they learned to cope, and what advice they would give to others going through it.

Sharing stories from real moms with Practical Advice

•Yasmin Regan, 33 years live in Australia/New York
Her Story with practical advice
"Having postpartum depression has been the most difficult thing I have ever experienced." I was completely miserable during a time when you are 'supposed' to be joyful.

When I was 30 weeks pregnant with my second child, who is now 15 months old, my first warning sign was intense rage. So it started with perinatal depression and progressed to postpartum depression. I recall being heavily pregnant and holding my toddler while my dog would not stop barking. The sound of his bark triggered something inside of me, and the next thing I knew, I was banging on our glass back door, which broke. I knew right away that something was seriously wrong.

"After those feelings of rage and overwhelm, I was suicidal by two weeks postpartum. My babies and husband, I was convinced, would be better off without me. I was exhausted from caring for a 16-month-old and a newborn. My husband works shifts, so I was often home alone with my children. I was filled with shame, guilt, and embarrassment. I had always wanted to be a mother, so I was perplexed as to why I was experiencing these symptoms.

I'm still going to therapy once a week, and I'm beginning a new antidepressant for the third time. The previous two didn't work. But, to be honest, talking about it on my Instagram page is the most cathartic for me. I document the ups and downs of having postpartum depression. I believe it is critical to surround myself with people who will not judge me. Many women suffer in silence. I also host the Mothering Through Postpartum Depression podcast.

Her Advice

My advice is that, no matter how embarrassed you are, there is no shame in what you are experiencing. There are many women who will understand how you feel. I wish I'd known it was more common than I thought and that I wasn't insane. We need more than a six-week check-up with a health worker: leaflets about postpartum depression and the risk factors for developing it should be available in every doctor's office."

•Linn-Beate S, 25years in Norway
Her Story with practical advice
"A large part of my postpartum depression was caused by our daughter's sleep regression at four months, which caused her to wake up at least once an hour to breastfeed." She was also struggling with the breast, which irritated me. My nights became sleepless, and I started to feel like the worst mother ever. I had a sense of helplessness, and I was afraid it would not go away. I'd read about a mother who came dangerously close to injuring her child, and I knew I was nowhere near that, but I was afraid of things getting worse. So I aware that I needed help. So I informed my partner and the healthcare provider. I felt a sense of relief the

moment I said it aloud. The next day, I spoke with my doctor online [due to COVID-19 restrictions], which was followed by a couple of sessions with a psychiatrist, who helped me with my mindset, most notably by telling me it would pass. I had my first session with a psychiatrist two days after asking for help. It could have been much worse if I had kept my emotions hidden. Inform people that it is normal to feel this way and that there is help available. It does not imply that you are a bad mother.

Her Advice

"I'd advise other mothers going through the same thing: it will pass." You will sleep again, and if you ask for help, you will be the best mother for your child."

•Rachael Phillipson, 29 years in UK
Her Story with practical advice
"It started while I was in the hospital with Lara, who was born six weeks premature. I remember crying in fear of her getting sick, thinking she

was infected and would die. My low mood and lack of emotions appeared to last longer than the typical 'baby blues' I'd experienced with my three older children. I felt completely dead inside, and nothing else mattered except protecting this baby.

"My relationship with my other children deteriorated. In the evenings, I'd sit in the bathroom and cry uncontrollably. My nightmares included my husband falling down the stairs while holding Lara and me pushing the pram into traffic. It was as if a voice told me to act on these dreams. I became suicidal, but I couldn't leave Lara behind because she needed me to breastfeed, so I felt compelled to bring her along.

"My husband had already noticed something was wrong and kept reminding me to talk to him about how I was feeling, so I told him. We then informed our health visitor, who notified my GP, who arranged for an emergency perinatal mental health nurse to visit me. She prescribed antidepressants for me.

"I found talking to the mental health nurse very helpful, and she helped me understand that, while having intrusive thoughts is frightening, they do not accurately reflect how I was feeling. She helped me feel understood and heard. My greatest fear of admitting how I felt was that my children would be taken away from me. I also had a nurse come in to help repair the bond with my older children, particularly my six-year-old daughter, who was the most affected.

"My husband was my biggest supporter. He encouraged me to go on walks to clear my mind and take care of myself. He also actively sought to develop a bond with Lara as my mind and mood improved. It's lovely to see his bond with her right now.

Her Advice

"My advice to new mothers is to educate themselves on postnatal depression during their pregnancy, and to get their fathers to do the same—just so you know what to look for. Also, if you are feeling low, talk to someone, anyone. The consequences of not talking about it and allowing your mind to go to the darkest of places can be devastating.

I wish I had known at the start of my depression that it is acceptable to be honest about how you feel; no one will judge you. "You are not a bad mother; you are human."

REVIEW

So with this book and all I can say is that this book is like a breath of fresh air for us new moms. It's like sitting with a friend and fully experiencing the range of emotions that come with the birth of a newborn.

The great thing is, it doesn't have to be difficult. The book contains practical advice that can be of help to all mothers. Whether you're a beginner or have been down this road before, there's something for everyone here.

And can we talk about these daily affirmations? A bonus section with 90 days of motivational quotes? Yes, please! It's the kind of little pick-me-up that any busy mom would appreciate.

The stories told in this book, combined with expert advice, easy self-care tips, and some great time management strategies, will help anyone feeling a little lost in the chaos of early birth. It's like having a friend who says, "It's okay if you don't understand everything right now." A companion for the days when you need wisdom, lots of encouragement, and a little help with postpartum issues. If you are a new mother or know someone who is, pick up this book. It's like a warm embrace for the soul in the midst of the beautiful chaos of motherhood. I will definitely recommend it.